HARNESSING THE HEALING POWER OF CRYST[AL]S
COLORING BOOK

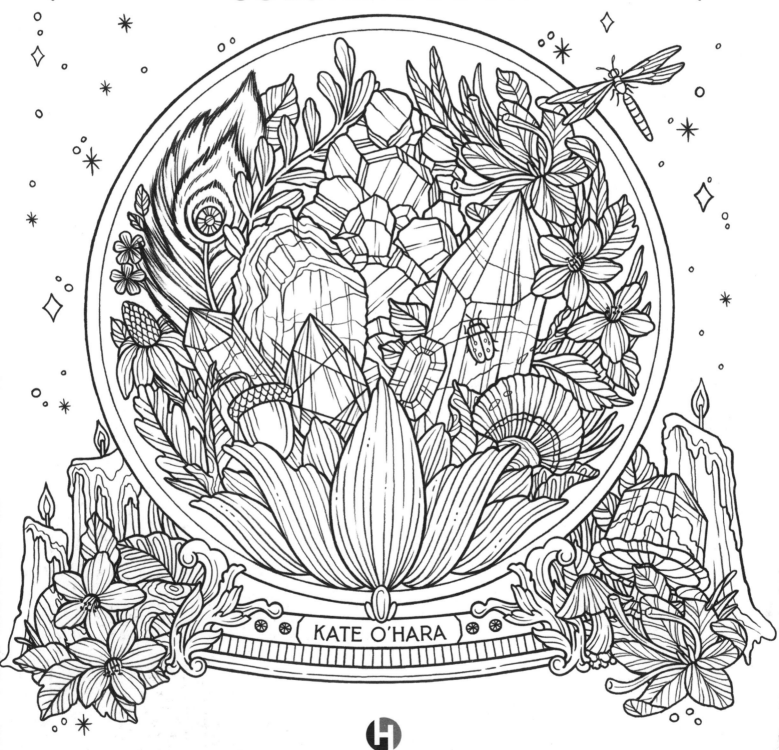

KATE O'HARA

HARVEST
An Imprint of WILLIAM MORROW

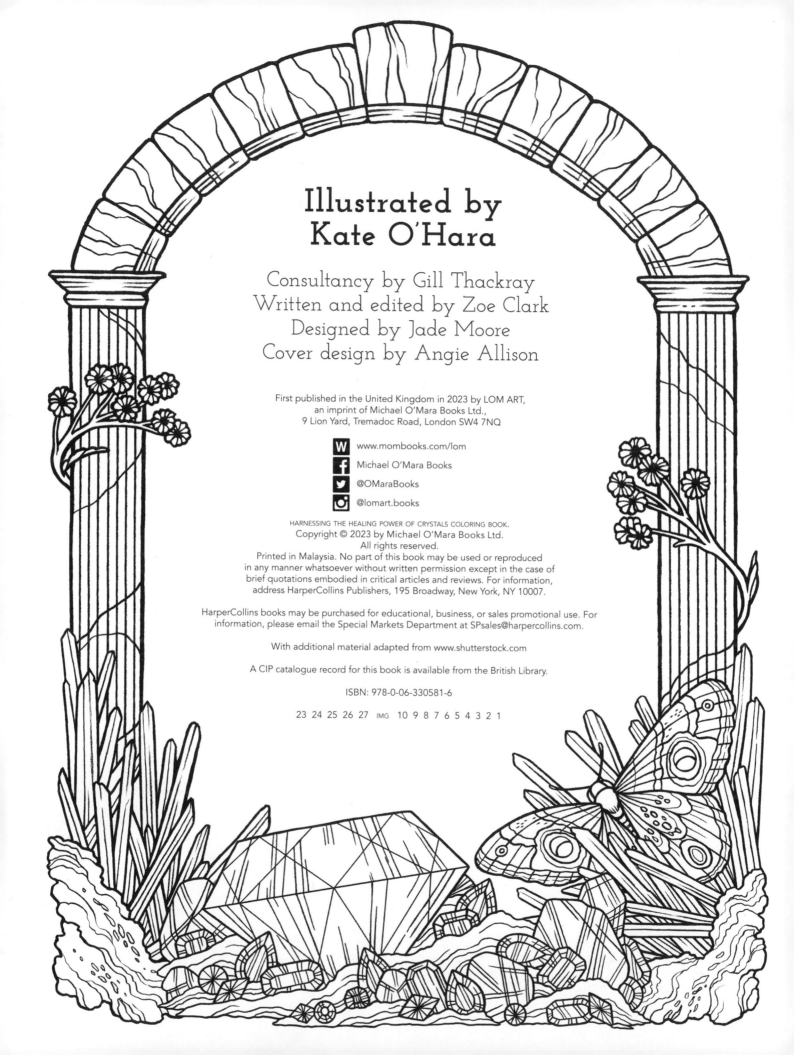

Illustrated by Kate O'Hara

Consultancy by Gill Thackray
Written and edited by Zoe Clark
Designed by Jade Moore
Cover design by Angie Allison

First published in the United Kingdom in 2023 by LOM ART,
an imprint of Michael O'Mara Books Ltd.,
9 Lion Yard, Tremadoc Road, London SW4 7NQ

W www.mombooks.com/lom
f Michael O'Mara Books
@OMaraBooks
@lomart.books

With additional material adapted from www.shutterstock.com

A CIP catalogue record for this book is available from the British Library.

ISBN: 978-0-06-330581-6

23 24 25 26 27 IMG 10 9 8 7 6 5 4 3 2 1

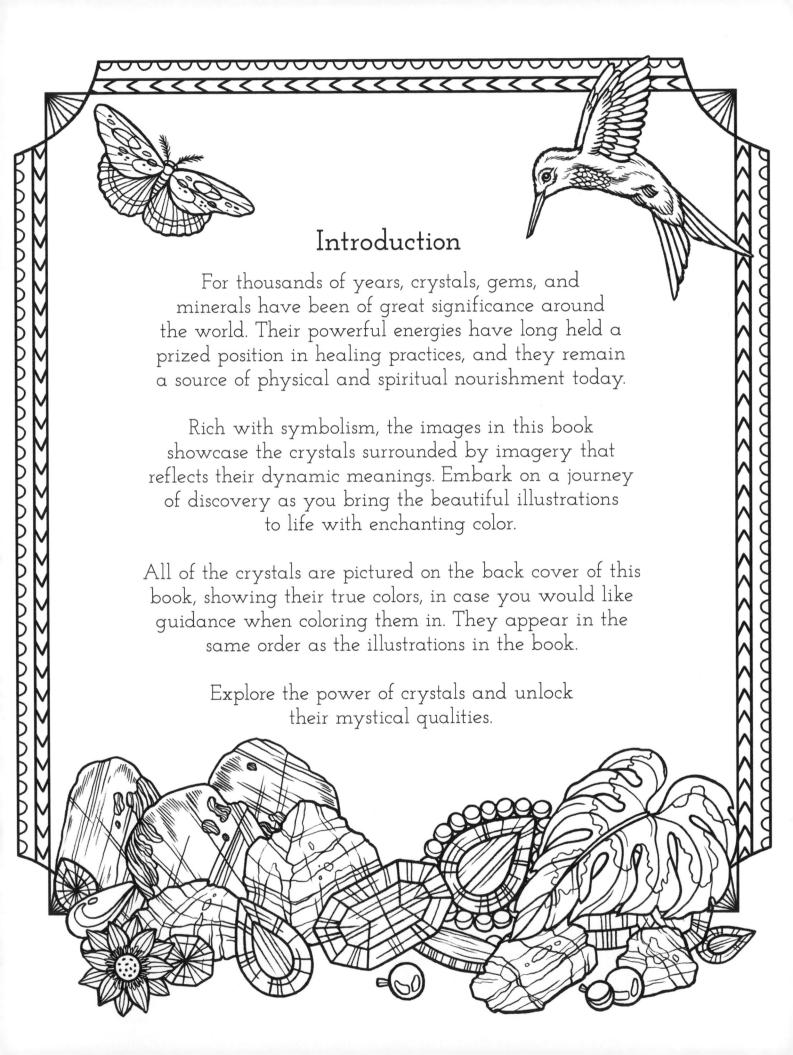

Introduction

For thousands of years, crystals, gems, and minerals have been of great significance around the world. Their powerful energies have long held a prized position in healing practices, and they remain a source of physical and spiritual nourishment today.

Rich with symbolism, the images in this book showcase the crystals surrounded by imagery that reflects their dynamic meanings. Embark on a journey of discovery as you bring the beautiful illustrations to life with enchanting color.

All of the crystals are pictured on the back cover of this book, showing their true colors, in case you would like guidance when coloring them in. They appear in the same order as the illustrations in the book.

Explore the power of crystals and unlock their mystical qualities.

A Note on Crystal Healing and Chakras

The word "chakra" comes from the word for "wheel" in Sanskrit, the sacred ancient language of Hinduism, and refers to centers of energy within the body. For thousands of years, societies all over the world have turned to the healing power of crystals to keep the body's chakra system in balance. There are seven main chakras which, when opened and aligned, are believed to allow energy to flow freely through the body.

Like all matter that makes up the universe, crystals carry unique energetic frequencies. Their vibrational energies are thought to transfer to the correlating chakra when held or placed near the body, returning these energetic centers to the frequencies they're meant to vibrate at and rebalancing any misalignment.

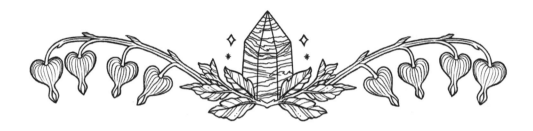

The **root chakra** is located at the base of the spine and is responsible for making you feel grounded, safe, and secure. It is associated with red and black crystals.

Beneath the belly button, the **sacral chakra** relates to our emotions and creative energies. Yellow and orange crystals are believed to activate the sacral chakra.

The **solar plexus chakra** is in the stomach area, and is associated with self-esteem and inner confidence. Crystals of yellow-golden hues often relate to this chakra.

Located in the chest, the **heart chakra** facilitates giving and receiving love, and encourages compassion and kindness. It is usually associated with green crystals.

Situated in the throat, the **throat chakra** relates to communication and self-expression, and is most commonly associated with blue crystals.

The **third eye chakra** is located between the eyebrows and governs intuition, wisdom, and imagination. Crystals that range in color from indigo to purple and blue relate to this chakra.

At the top of the head, the **crown chakra** represents spiritual connections to higher realms of consciousness. Most crystals that connect to the crown chakra are purple.

Colored by

....

Amber

Associated with relieving anxiety and improving
self-esteem, amber can help to ward off negativity
and bring a bright, calming energy in its place.
Typically honey-yellow in color with a golden
glow that captures the warmth of the Sun, amber
represents positivity and renewal.

Amber is formed from the fossilized resin of pine trees,
meaning it is deeply imbued with the life force from
prehistoric forests, preserving their ancient wisdom.

Across mythologies, amber has always held a strong
connection to the Sun, Earth, and animal kingdom.
Believing that amber contained the wisdom and strength
of animals, the Vikings carved pieces of amber resin into
beautiful jewelry, tools, and protective amulets,
like the bear carving pictured here.

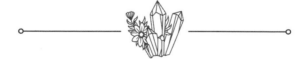

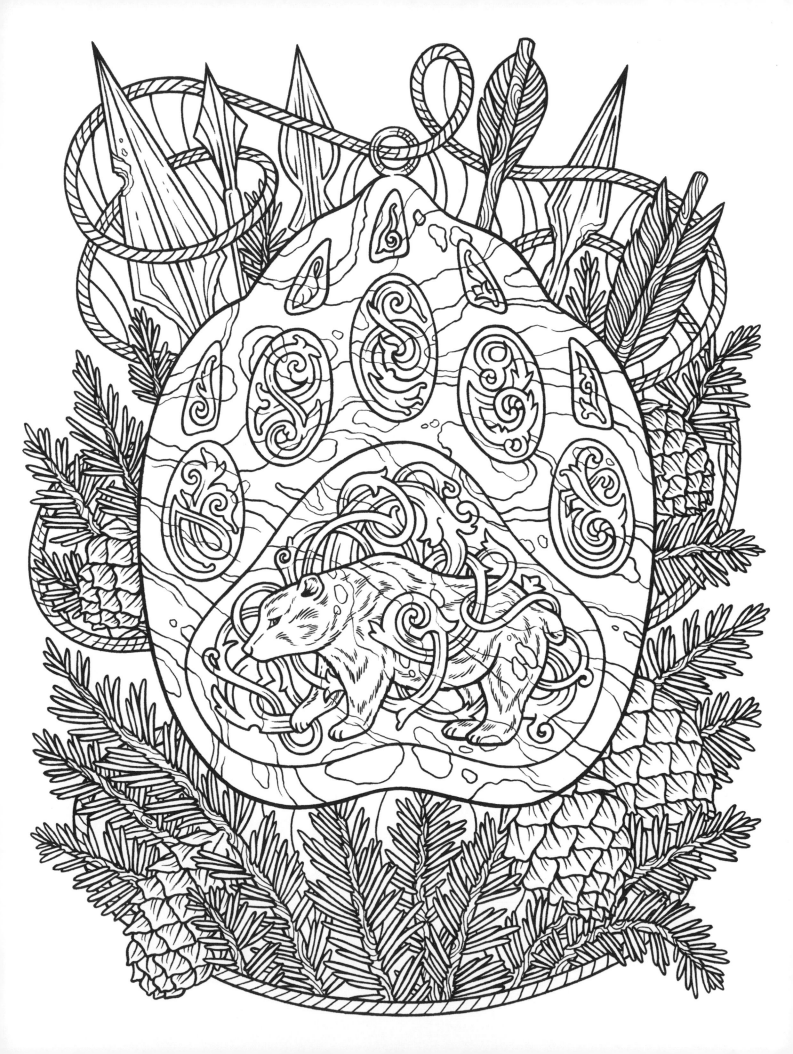

Kammererite

Deep-purple hues associated with the crown chakra are fused with the soothing green shades of the heart chakra in this highly intuitive crystal. The result is a beautiful stone with a connection to the higher self and the power to cultivate emotional balance and prosperity.

The heart-based energy of kammererite means it has excellent emotional healing properties. Many believe it can be used to open the mind to new experiences and nurture relationships, inviting eternal joy and happiness into the user's life.

A stone of true kindness and generosity, it is thought to guide a person's moral compass, steering them towards compassion, warmth, and understanding for those around them.

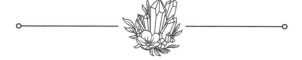

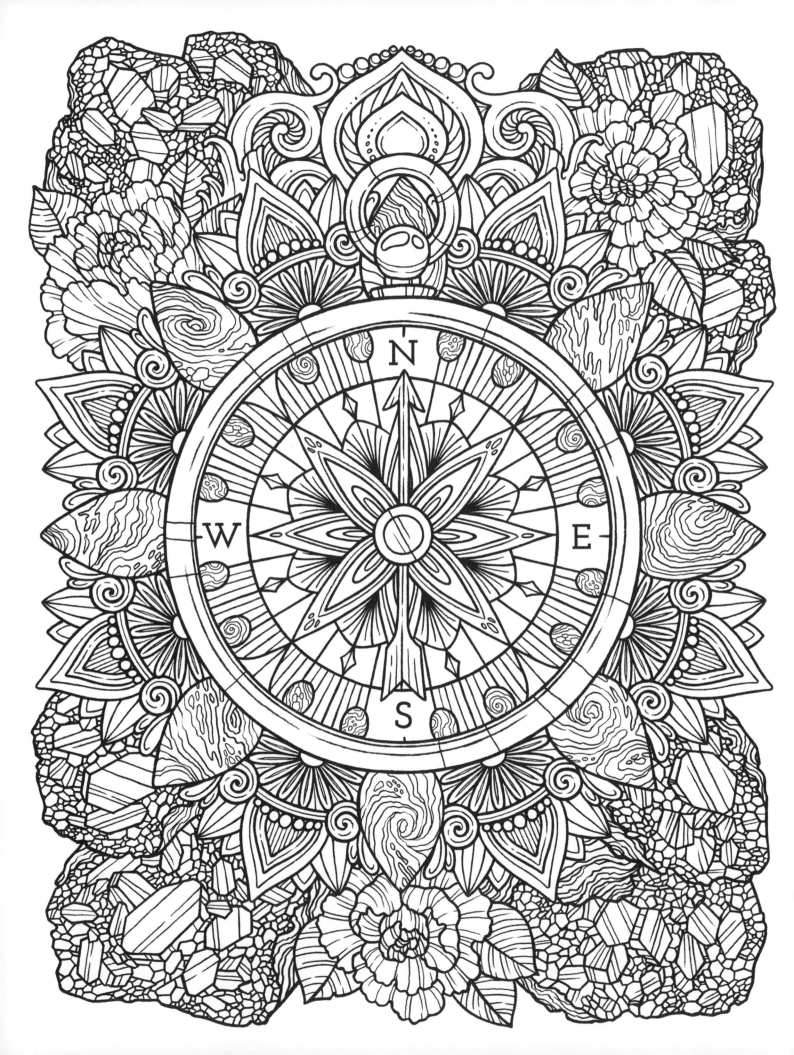

Azurite

Azurite has an enchanting, swirling pattern made
up of energetic and vivid blues, ranging from midnight
to azure. Believed to be one of the most potent psychic
stones, azurite has been held in high spiritual
reverence for thousands of years.

Across ancient cultures, azurite was considered a
sacred stone with intense spiritual healing abilities.
It was believed to have the power to open celestial
gateways in ancient China. Native Americans used it
for communication with spirit guides and it was prized
among high priests and priestesses in ancient Egypt.

Today, it is still profoundly connected to inner wisdom,
intuition, and psychic awareness, much like the crystal
ball pictured here. Helping to cleanse the aura and realign
all the chakras, this alluring stone is overflowing
with spiritual and visionary powers.

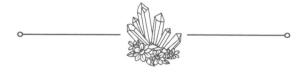

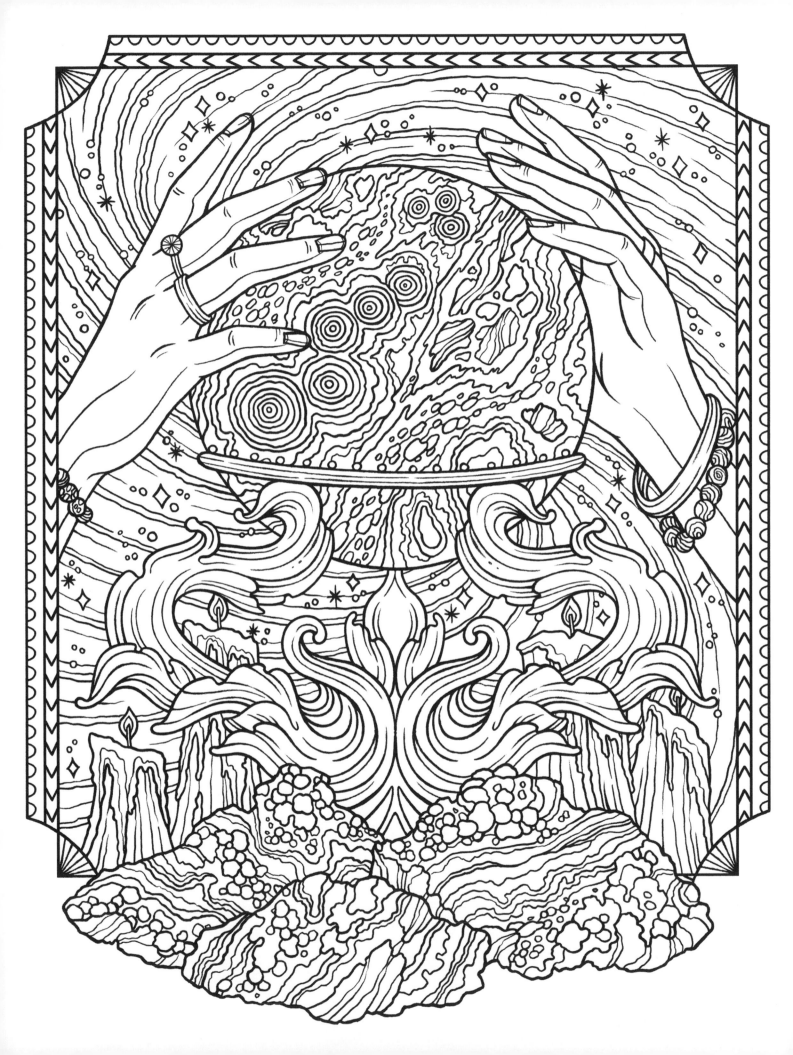

Pyrite

This dazzling stone is fiercely bold with its
glistening golden hues and bright metallic luster.
It is also known as fool's gold, thanks to its bright
and brassy resemblance to gold.

Pyrite is associated with abundance and prosperity,
and its energies protect the possessor from all forms
of negativity. With a strong connection to the solar
plexus and sacral chakras, it is thought to increase
creativity, confidence, and willpower.

Pyrite takes its name from the Greek word for fire.
If struck hard enough, it will create sparks, a property
which signifies its potent protective powers, like a dragon
shielding its treasures. Synonymous with the flames of a
blazing fire, this stone inspires passion and determination.

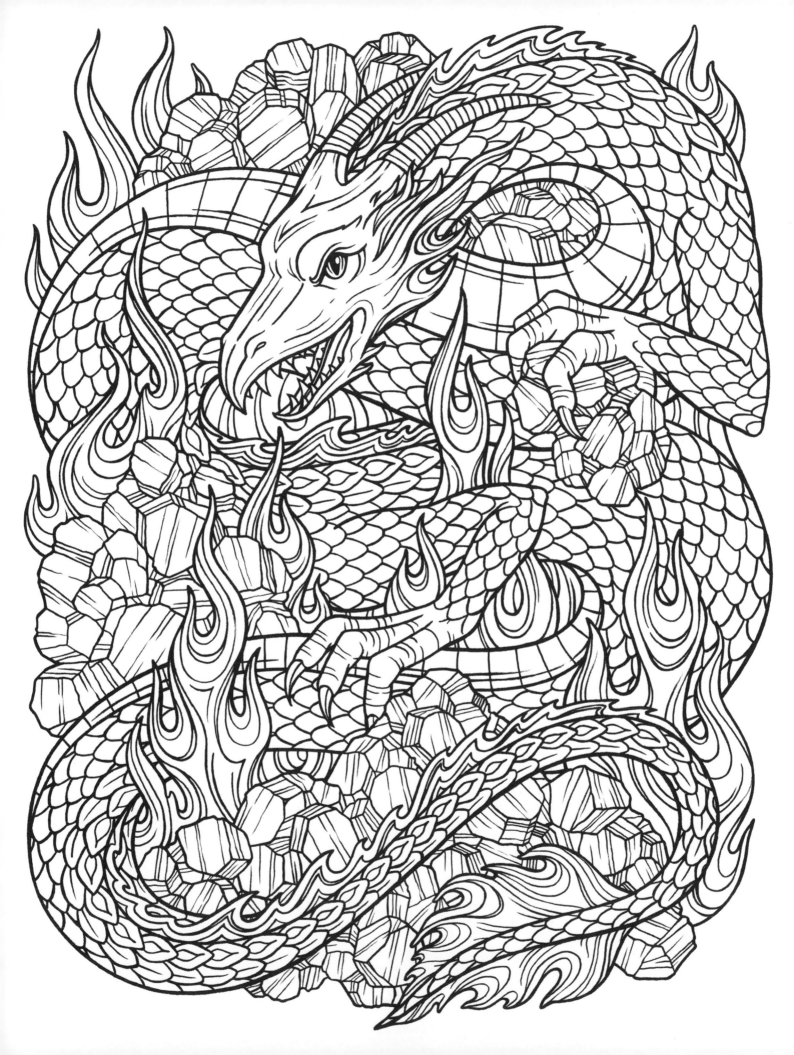

Angelite

Said to be the crystal of angels, angelite is
associated with mindfulness, protection, and peace.
Holding this stone close to the heart is thought to help bring
spiritual guidance from higher realms of consciousness.
A powerful communication stone, it is believed to
assist with self-expression and lucid dreaming.

Calming and soothing, angelite comes in the
sky-blue hues of a clear, cloudless day. Its soft, tranquil
nature and ethereal energies are believed to dispel anger
and anxiety, boosting the mood and leaving a
feeling of pure and perfect serenity.

Here, a heart-shaped angelite stone is adorned
with a beautiful halo and angel wings. Surrounded by
an elegant wreath of angel's breath and daisies, the stone
is pictured high among the clouds, synonymous with
its celestial and peaceful properties.

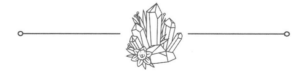

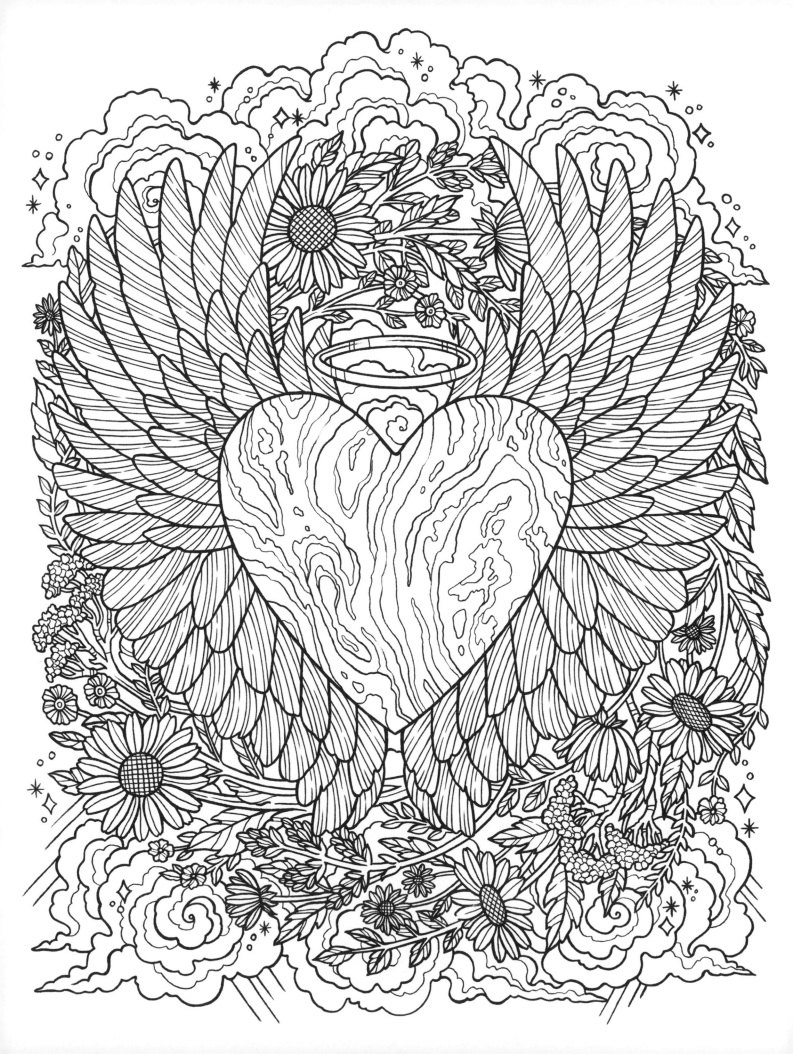

Black Tourmaline

This inky stone acts as a shield of protection, strength, and self-confidence. It was often used by ancient magicians during rituals to ward off demonic forces and evil spirits. Still revered today for its deeply protective powers, it allows its owner to overcome setbacks and dispel negative thought patterns, attracting positive energies in their place.

With a strong connection to the root chakra, black tourmaline is primarily a grounding stone. Like a sturdy oak tree anchored to the ground with its winding roots, it symbolizes stability and security. The black cat pictured here is symbolic of spiritual protection, and this potent stone of purification has the ability to transform toxic energies into something positive. This allows the possessor to feel safe and nurtured, as if wrapped in a cloak of protection.

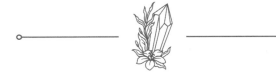

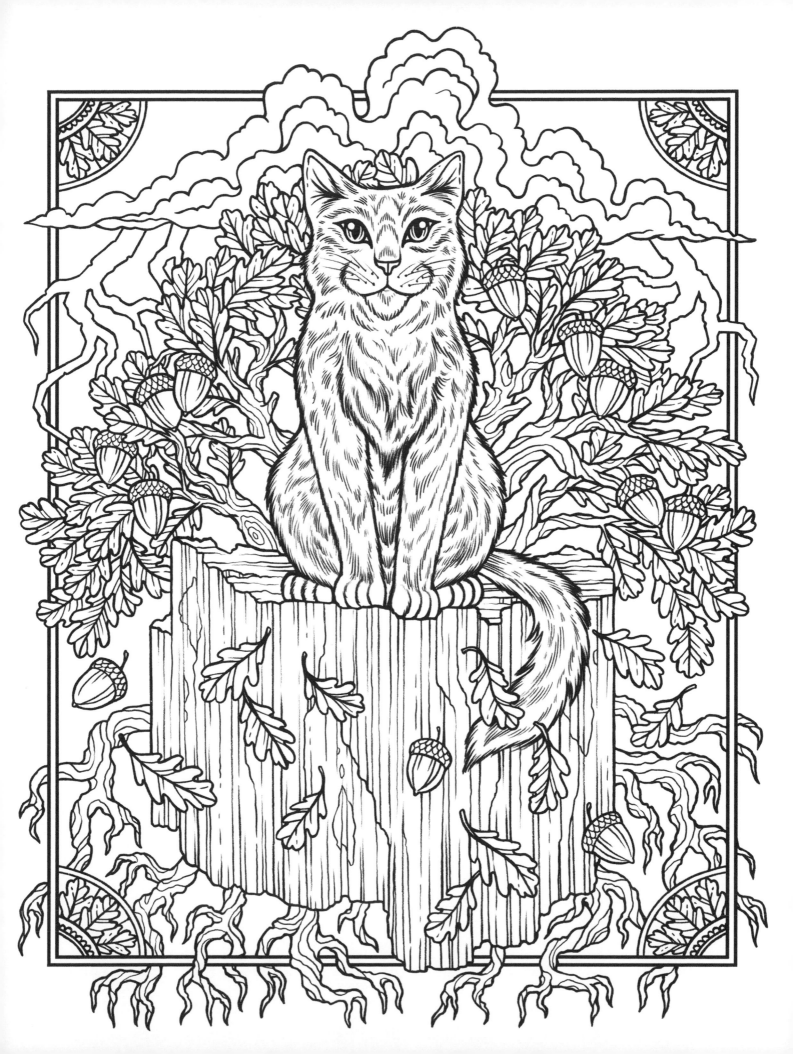

Morganite

Soft and sweet, the peachy-pink hues of morganite
echo its association with innocence, romance, and love.
Imitating the calming colors of a hazy sunrise, this is a
stone of divine love, which helps to nurture connections
and improve communication with loved ones.

Closely connected with the heart chakra, morganite
is thought to invite emotional healing and to help
overcome fear and resentment. Believed to stimulate
an open and energized heart, this compassionate
crystal can help with all matters of the heart, from
attracting a soulmate and cherishing existing
relationships to mending a broken heart.

Here, the crystal is shown with a pair of lovebirds,
the picture of everlasting devotion, and an array
of luscious fruit and delicate flowers, symbolic
of passion, femininity, and romance.

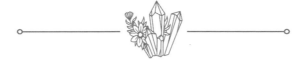

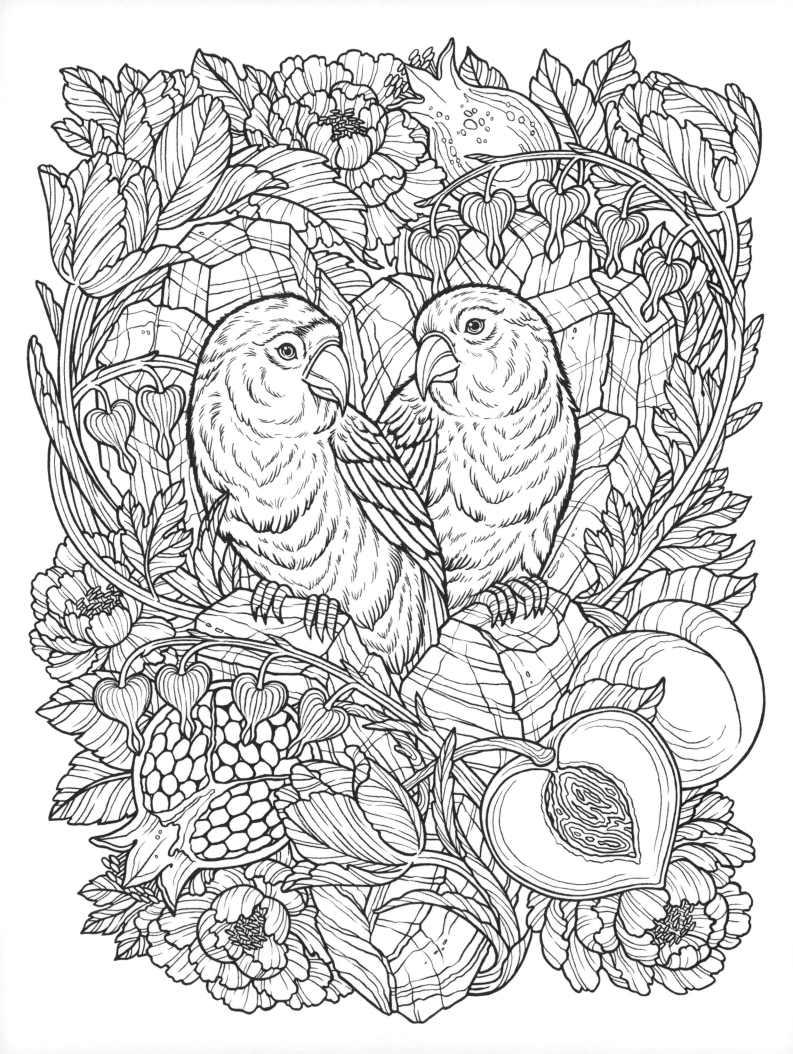

Selenite

Named after the Greek goddess of the Moon, selenite is primarily a stone of protection and is associated with the divine feminine and lunar energies. Often found in soft and serene shades of silvery, luminous white, it holds a soothing power, evoking the tranquility of the Moon glowing in the night sky. Thought to have cleansing and rejuvenating abilities, this mystical stone offers gentle guidance in times of transition.

Here, selenite towers are surrounded by the swirling waves of a swelling tide, and by wolves, which symbolize the wild and powerful nature of womanhood. The Moon's phases represent the rhythm of life and the cycles of nature. Selenite invites its possessor to connect with this cosmic rhythm, and to feel in tune with the ebb and flow of the world's natural energies.

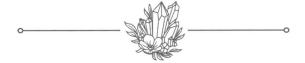

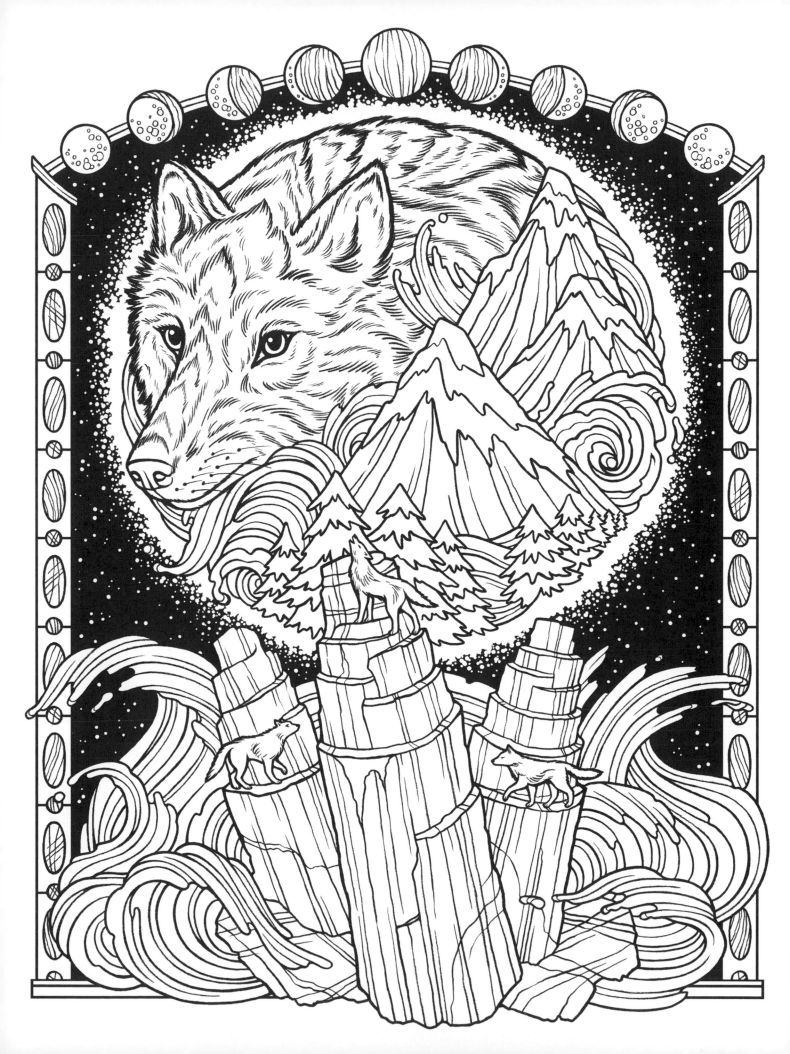

Emerald

This revitalizing gemstone has been prized
throughout history as a stone of compassion and romance.
The enchanting green hues of emerald mean it is profoundly
linked to the heart chakra, helping its wearer experience
eternal and unconditional divine love.

Emerald is soothing and stimulating in equal measure,
with its calming green tones and shimmering luster.
It has carried the meaning of rebirth and eternal life
since antiquity, and today it remains a gemstone
used to promote vivacious health.

The tree of life and ancient ouroboros symbols shown
here are rich with spiritual meaning, representing the
balance and unity of all living things and the eternal
cycle of life. The gemstone of spring, renewal, and new
beginnings, emerald evokes this same spiritual meaning,
bringing harmonious energy to all aspects of life.

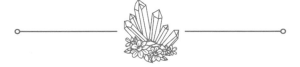

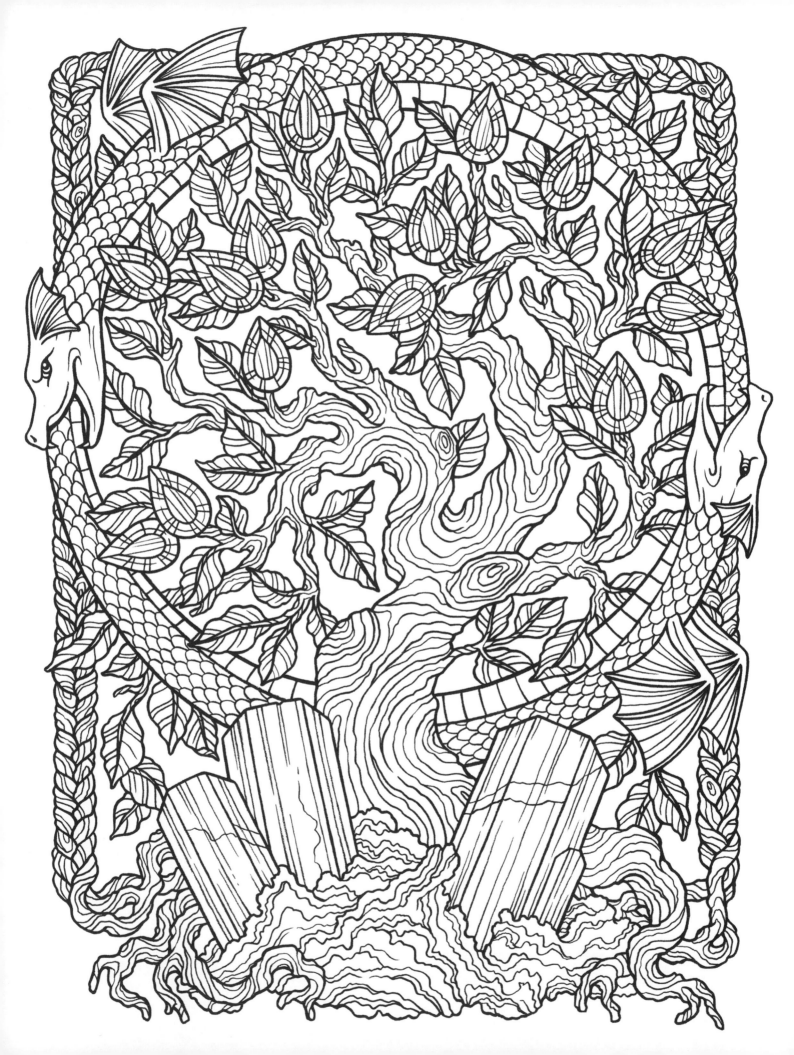

Citrine

Believed to hold the energy of the Sun, citrine is a
powerful stone of imagination, self-expression, and creativity.
With a warm and citrus-colored appearance, varying
from pale-yellow to burnt-orange shades, it encourages
optimism and happiness, bringing a positive
flow of energy to the body.

This "Sun stone" uplifts the spirit and cultivates confidence.
It is said to bring success and prosperity, with many
believing it attracts wealth and fortune. This makes it
the perfect stone to assist in manifesting financial and
spiritual abundance. Opening the solar plexus chakra,
citrine facilitates new beginnings while encouraging
clarity of thinking and emotional well-being.

Here, it is set within the petals of a sunflower and
between rays of glorious sunlight. Both are common
symbols of happiness, healing, and protection, much
like this powerful and positive crystal.

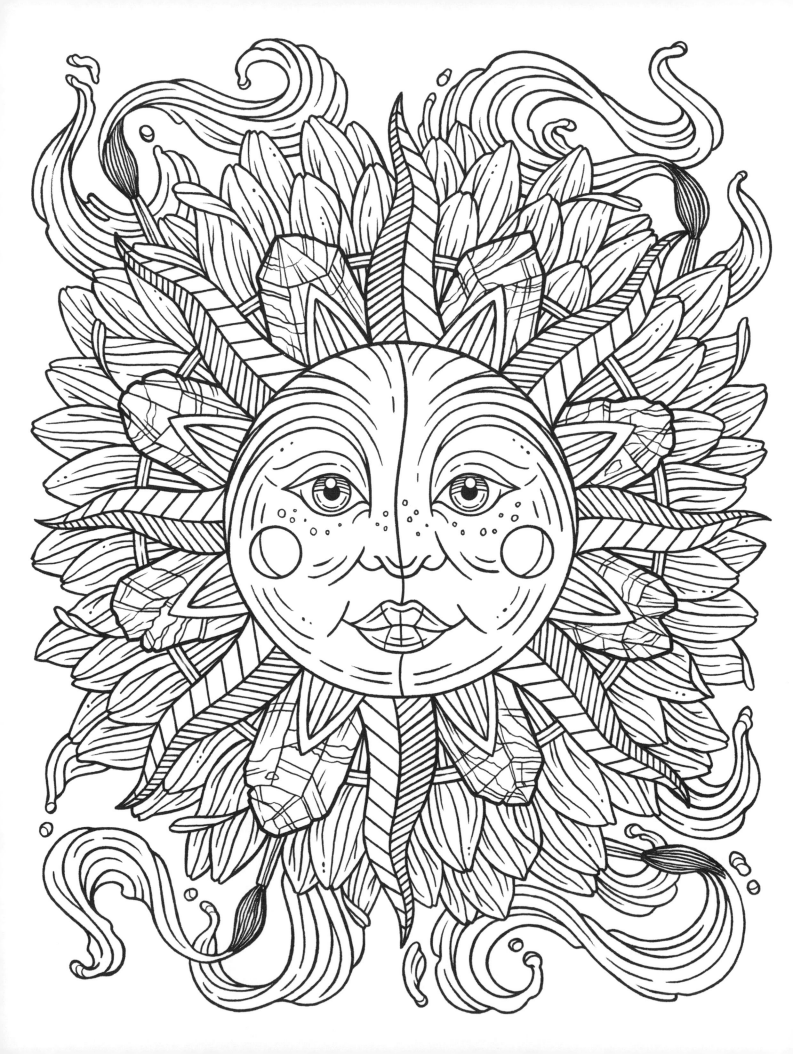

Aquamarine

Aquamarine ranges from paler hues to deep
and dazzling shades of blue. Closely associated with the
ocean, its mesmerizing and soothing appearance evokes
the tranquility of crystalline waters. Possessing the
cleansing energy of the sea, this crystal represents
purity, healing, and harmony.

In ancient times, the stone was thought to be
the treasure of mermaids. It was said to protect sailors
from rough seas and bring them safely back to land
through calm waves. Still believed to protect travelers
today, aquamarine remains a symbol of hope
and courage for many people.

By opening the channels of clear and heartfelt
communication, aquamarine is said to increase sensitivity
and sharpen the senses. The stone of cleansing and openness,
it can bring peace and clarity to those who use it.

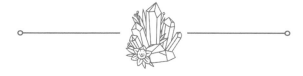

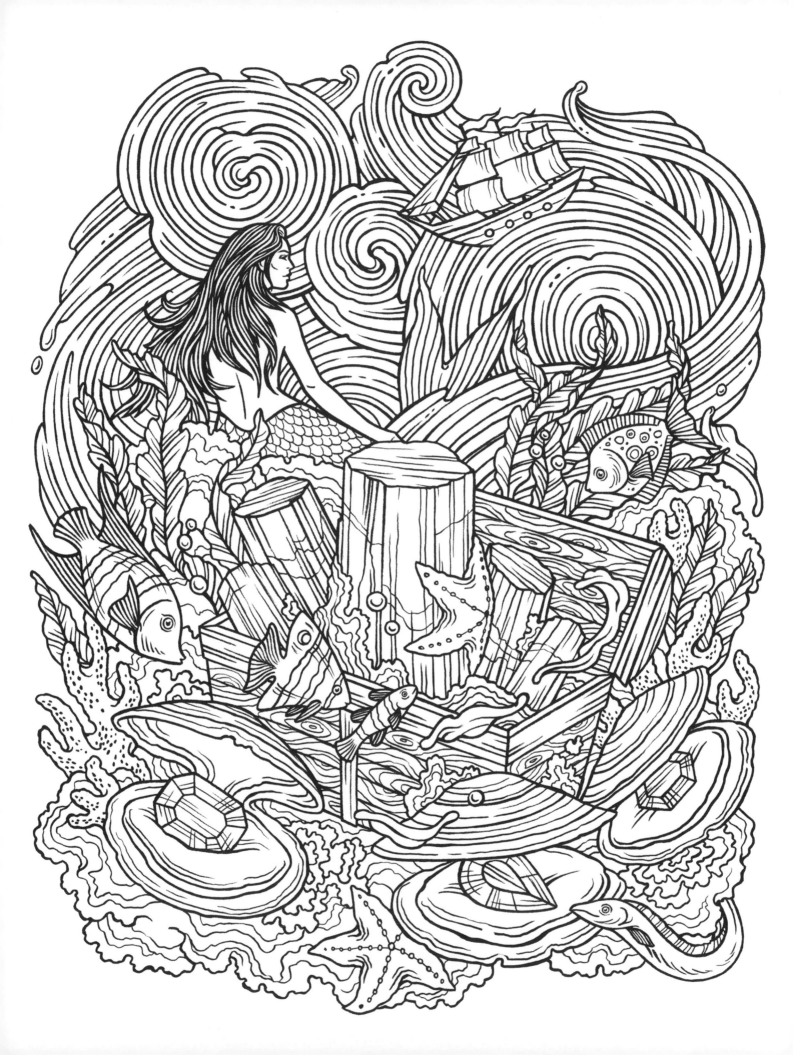

Ruby

For thousands of years, ruby has been prized as a stone
of romantic love, passion, and sensuality. Its deep and alluring
red coloring and its rich, glowing hues give the precious
gemstone its historic connections to wealth, power, and
nobility in cultures throughout the world.

Like a light that shines in the darkness, ruby
inspires a sense of power in the possessor, encouraging
self-confidence and determination. By stimulating a flow
of energy to the root chakra, ruby helps to bring about
vitality, spiritual wellness, and a lust for life.

Here, the gemstone is pictured burning brightly
within a bejeweled lantern, alluding to its regal reputation
throughout history. The ruby fireflies are also emitting
a glowing light, representing the illuminated, clear
mind and impassioned spirit that ruby enables.

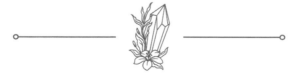

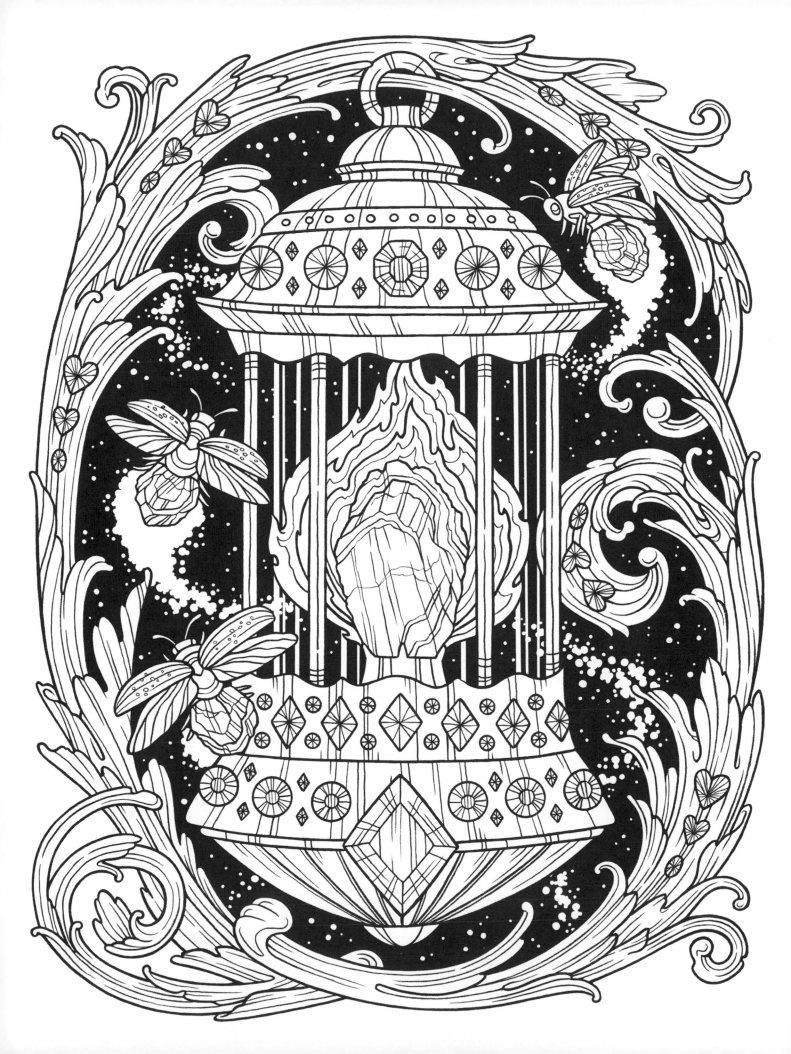

Howlite

Pearly white streaked with dark, silvery veins,
howlite is a soothing stone in both appearance
and nature. Bringing patience and perspective, it
is believed to encourage emotional expression,
eliminate anger, and steady a busy mind.

Like the rolling waves and sea breeze on a sunny
day, howlite invites its possessor to find a sense of calm
during times of stress. Here, howlite stones adorn the
surface of a beautiful conch shell and are tumbling
freely from it. The conch shell is believed to be a
symbol of protection and purification with
a strong connection to the dream world.

With an attunement to the Divine and a close
connection to the crown chakra, many people believe
howlite aids connections to higher truth and wisdom.

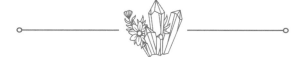

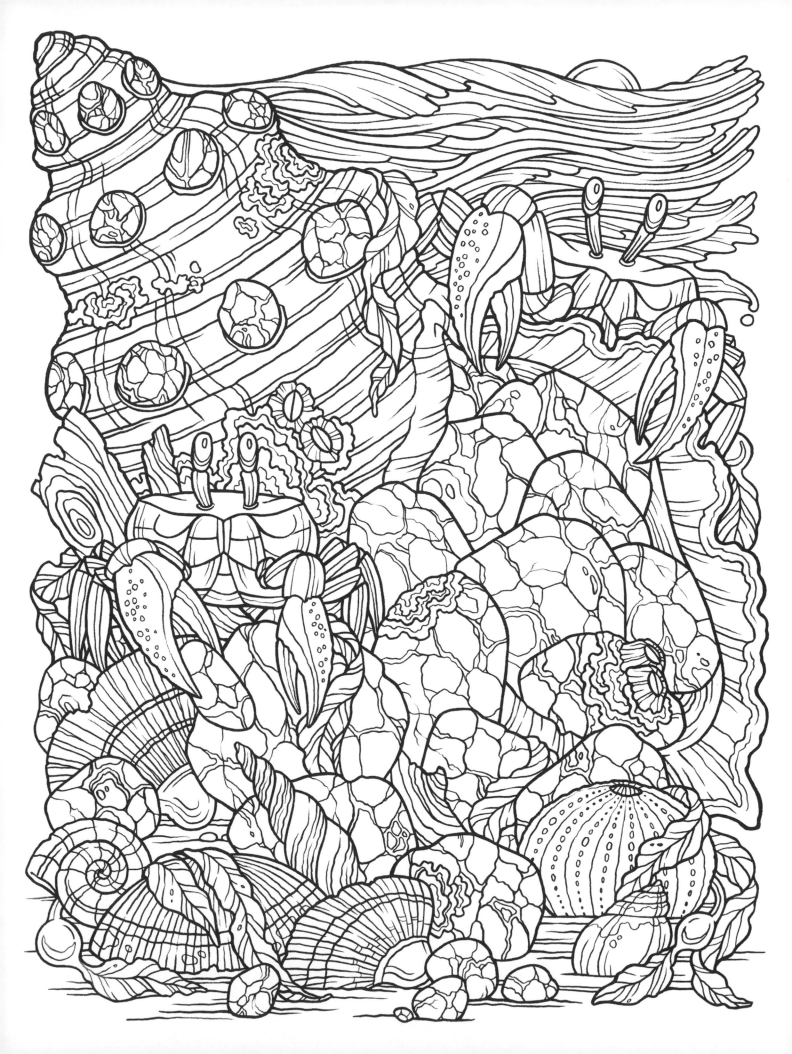

Scolecite

Scolecite is a deeply restorative crystal with high-frequency vibrations, meaning its powerful energies can be used to strengthen meditative states and assist lucid dreaming. Formed in clusters of sharp, needle-like points and most commonly found in exquisite tones of moonlight bluish-white, it is a powerful stone of inter-dimensional awareness and spiritual transformation.

Known as the stone of inner peace, scolecite has a particular affinity with the crown and third eye chakras. It invites possessors to find enlightenment and expand their consciousness into the spirit realm.

Here, the crystal is pictured within a mystical woodland scene in the deep of night. With powers of wisdom and intuition, the owl has long been a symbol of independent thinking and supernatural foresight. Scolecite is believed to equip the user with the same sharpness and strength of mind as this wise and mysterious creature.

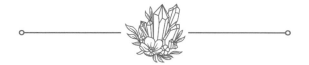

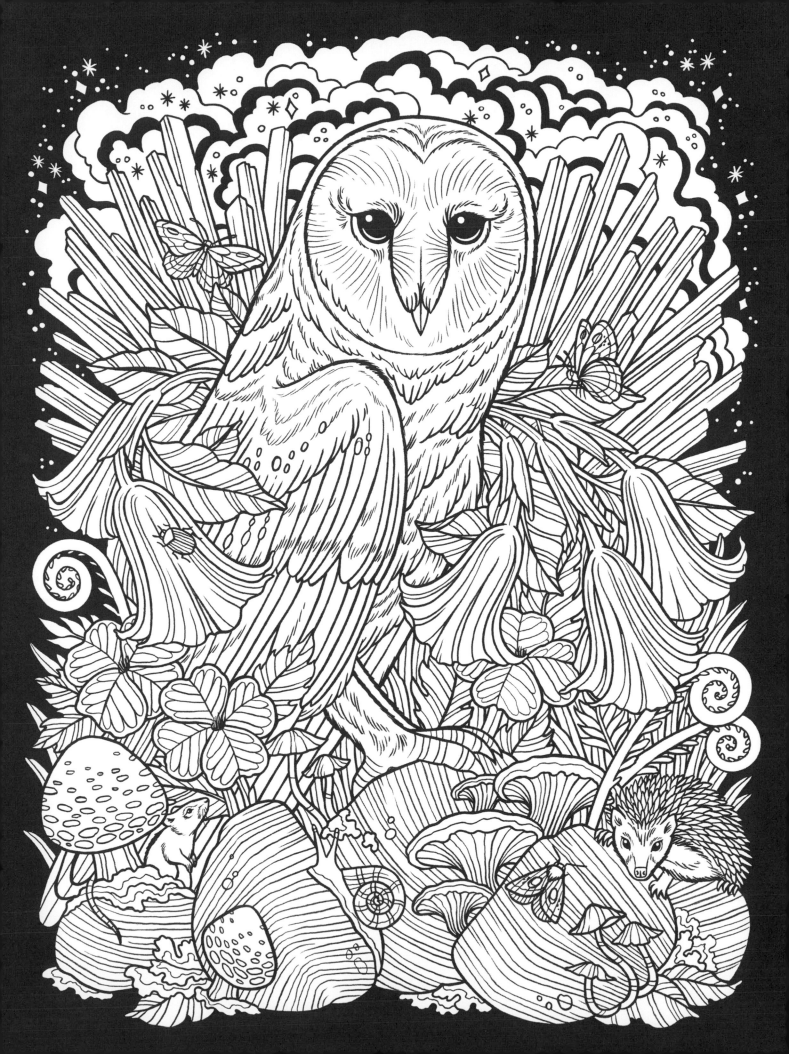

Crocoite

Crocoite is named after the ancient Greek word
for saffron due to its intense orange-red color. It is made
up of overlapping shards of vibrant red crystal in a
striking and unique formation. Here, the crystals appear
to be blooming from the center of saffron crocus flowers,
interspersed with the real saffron stigmas from
which their name is derived.

Crocoite is known as the "breakthrough stone" for its
transformative and supportive energies that aid a person
in times of transition. The butterflies throughout this image
carry the same symbolic meaning. A highly energetic
stone, it enhances creativity and encourages free-flowing
ideas, like the rushing waters of a river.

Unlocking and linking the root, heart, and crown
chakras, this powerful stone works to instill energy and
vitality throughout the whole body, bringing powerful
emotional and mental healing.

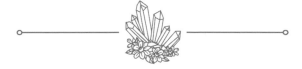

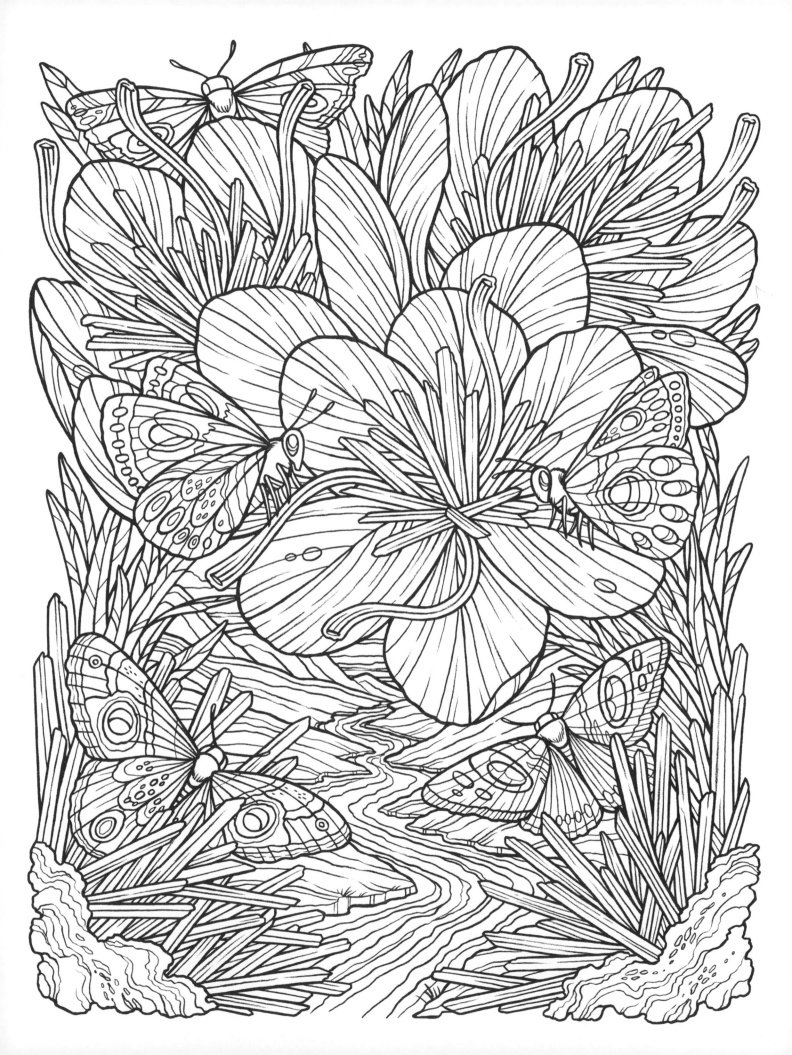

Jet

Formed from the wood of ancient trees, jet is a grounding stone that connects its wearer to the Earth's energies through the root chakra. It is a highly protective stone, and has been used throughout history to shield the possessor from negativity and deflect the "evil eye," a malevolent gaze thought to bring harm.

Here, polished jet stones are enveloped by tree roots, evoking the sense of stability jet provides, and the winding snakes symbolize healing. A universal symbol of protection, the Hamsa Hand is thought to bring happiness, health, and good fortune, like the expansive energies of this stone.

With an enchanting color of the deepest black, jet is associated with purity and detoxification. This sleek stone cleanses the aura, removing toxicity and channeling it into dynamic, productive energy.

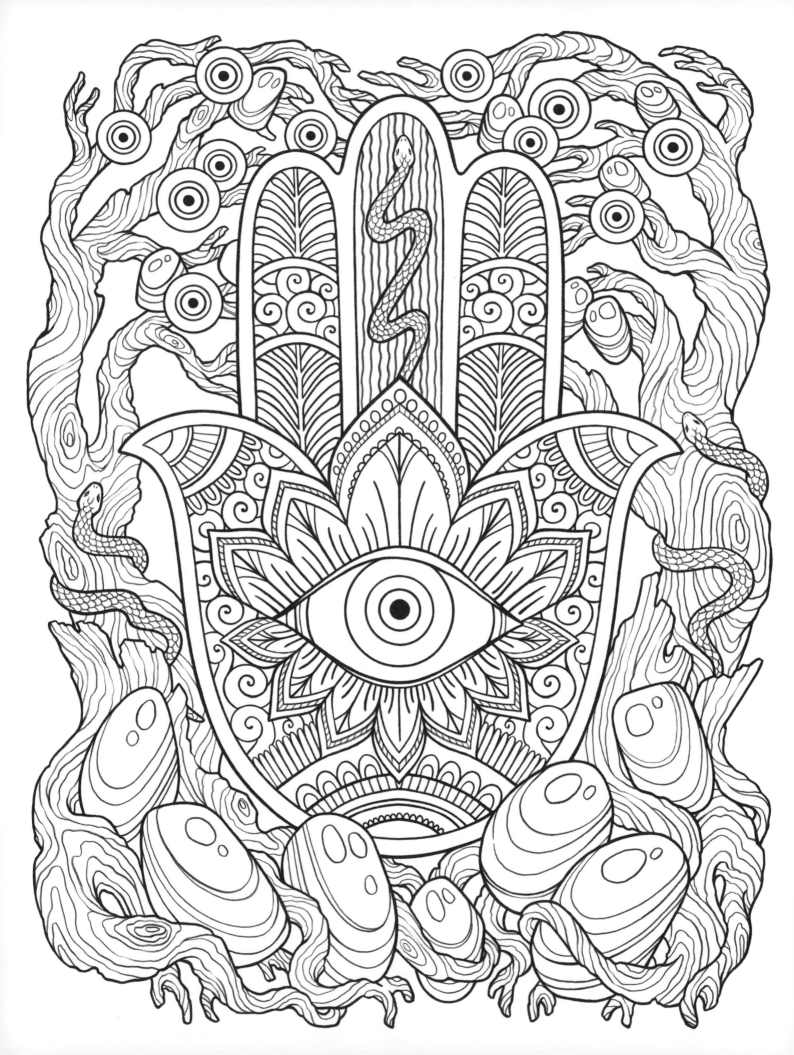

Rainbow Fluorite

Also known as the "genius stone," this captivating crystal encourages clarity of thinking, and inspires deep focus and productivity. It comes in an array of colors, with mesmerizing stripes formed from the purple, green, blue, and yellow varieties of fluorite. Simultaneously promoting a sense of calm while radiating creative energies, it brings joy and harmony while sweeping away negativity.

Rainbow fluorite is a powerful crystal for cleansing the chakras, as each color connects to a different chakra. With purple shades stimulating the third eye, green hues opening the heart, and deep blues activating the throat chakra, this vibrant crystal provides a deep sense of realignment throughout the whole body.

Taking its name from the Latin word for flux, rainbow fluorite helps its possessor flow freely from one state of being to another—with balance and positivity—just as the icy branches of winter give way to the full bloom of summer. Like a rainbow in the sky, this energizing crystal refreshes the mind and revitalizes the soul.

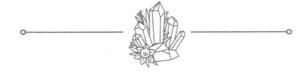

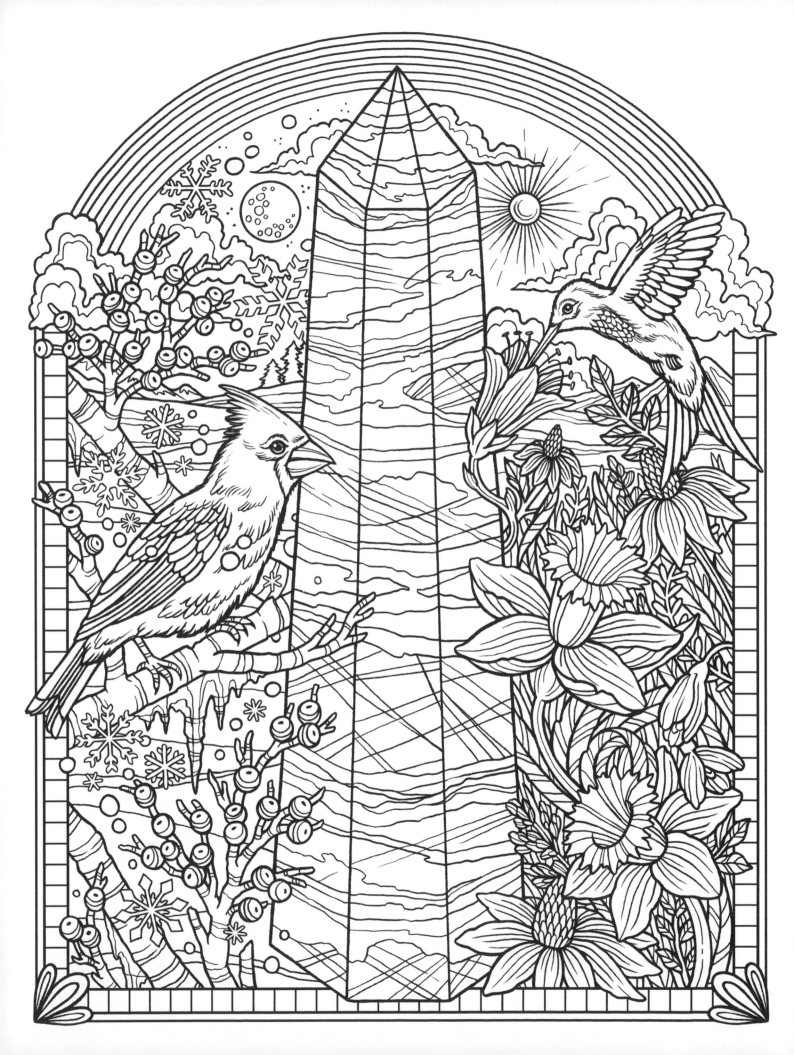

Jade

Most often associated with cool and calming
shades of green, jade promotes serenity and harmony.
Synonymous with the healing powers of Mother Earth,
this soothing stone nurtures the mind and soul, and brings
balance to the body. Jade is associated with purity
and wisdom, and many people believe it facilitates
moral integrity and prosperity.

Revered as the most precious stone in ancient China,
jade was often carved into ornaments, jewelry, and
tools, adorned with beautiful designs and thought to protect
and purify their users. Much like the crystal itself, the
tortoise shown here is a strong symbol of endurance, luck,
and longevity in feng shui, the Chinese practice of creating
a harmonious space to promote success, balance, and
happiness. The sturdy shell of the tortoise invokes
jade's protective power to provide a long and
prosperous life to those who use it.

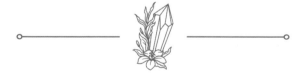

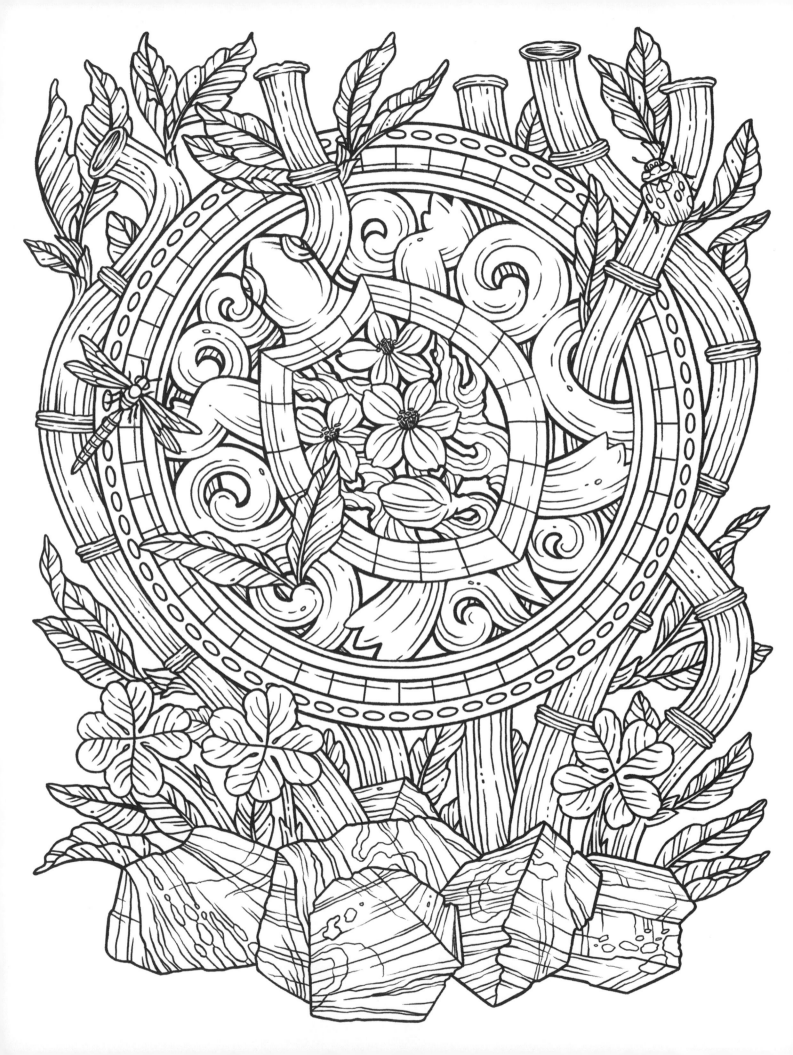

Amethyst

A symbol of peace and serenity, amethyst is
deeply connected to spiritual healing and purification.
Its beautiful, mystical purple color, ranging from light
lavender to vivid violet shades, is linked to deepening
awareness and enhancing insight and wisdom.

Amethyst is closely connected to the third eye
chakra, helping to awaken intuition and guide the
owner on their spiritual path. The crystal is pictured here
amidst the petals of a lotus flower, and is accompanied
by intuitive, all-seeing butterflies. It is an image of
true tranquility, rich with the symbolism of
transformation and spiritual awakening.

Soothing and uplifting, this is an empowering
stone that helps its possessor gain a greater sense of
understanding about their place in the world.
It facilitates embracing new challenges with
an open and clear mind.

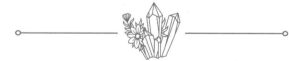

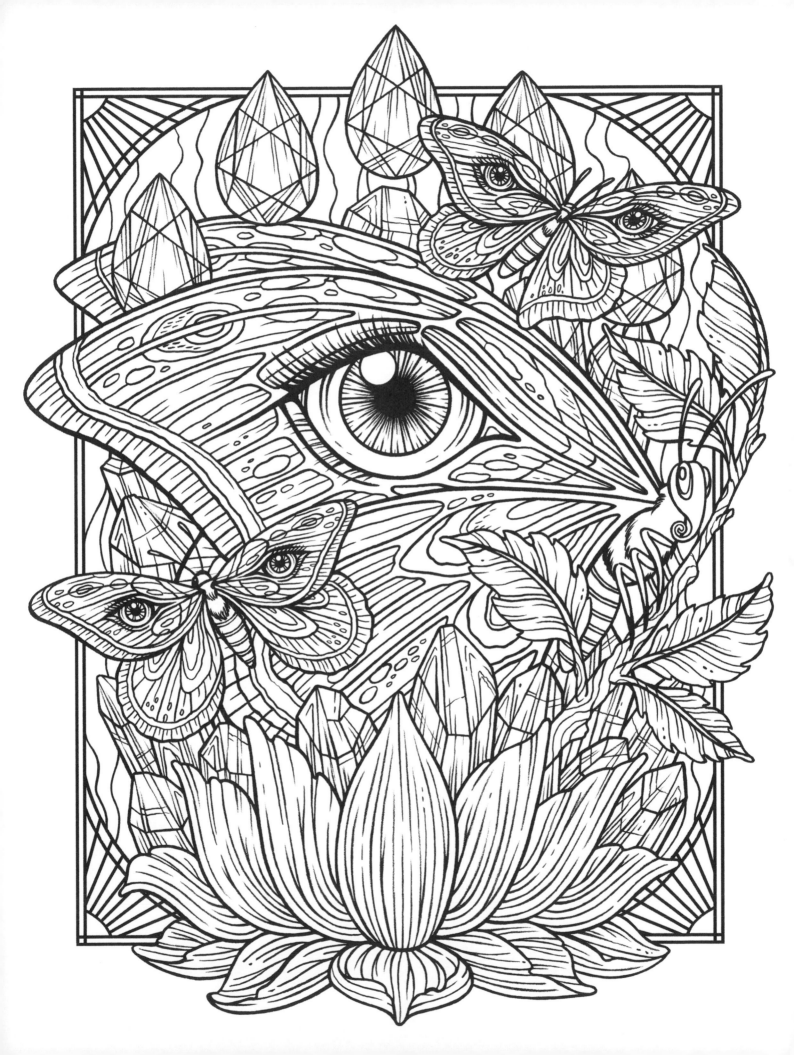

Desert Rose

Desert rose crystals are highly spiritual stones
with strong metaphysical powers. They are intricate,
rose-like formations shaped by the elements in arid climates.
Ranging from creamy white to dark beige in color,
they carry a powerful vibrational energy which is said
to strengthen our connection to higher realms.

The appeal of this crystal lies not only in its unique
appearance, but also in its divine qualities, which assist in
manifestation and achieving mental clarity. It is thought
to unlock the dreams and desires of the higher self.

Here, a cluster of desert rose crystals is shown among
the blossoming flowers of a desert rose plant. It is believed
that every desert rose crystal holds a "spirit guardian"
and provides a bridge between Heaven and Earth, like
a beautiful horizon at sunset where mountains
meet the skies above.

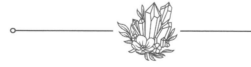

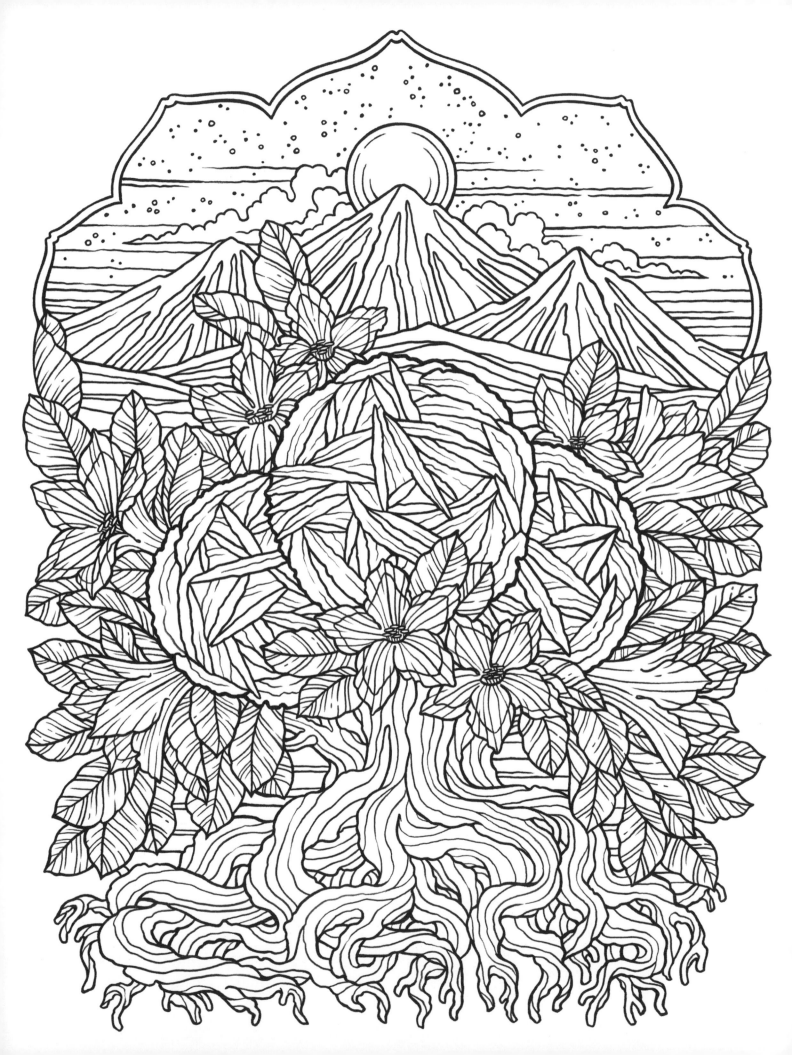

Rose Quartz

Known as the "heart stone," rose quartz comes in a
spectrum of colors synonymous with romance, from
the palest of blush pinks to deep and vibrant violet.
With a delicacy of appearance that belies its strength,
this is the crystal of universal and unconditional love.

Here, the gem is accompanied by roses, a symbol of
love and beauty, and a clutch of heart-shaped strawberries.
The interlocking pair of flamingos echoes the delicate pink
coloring of the crystal. Rose quartz invites compassion and
care, and encourages emotional connection on all levels.
It can be used to help attract new love, reinforce
family ties, or nurture friendships.

Rose quartz is deeply connected to the heart chakra,
and can help to heal emotional wounds. No one is immune
to Cupid's arrow, and this stone can be a powerful force for
those who desire more love in their lives, whether from
external relationships or from within.

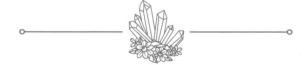

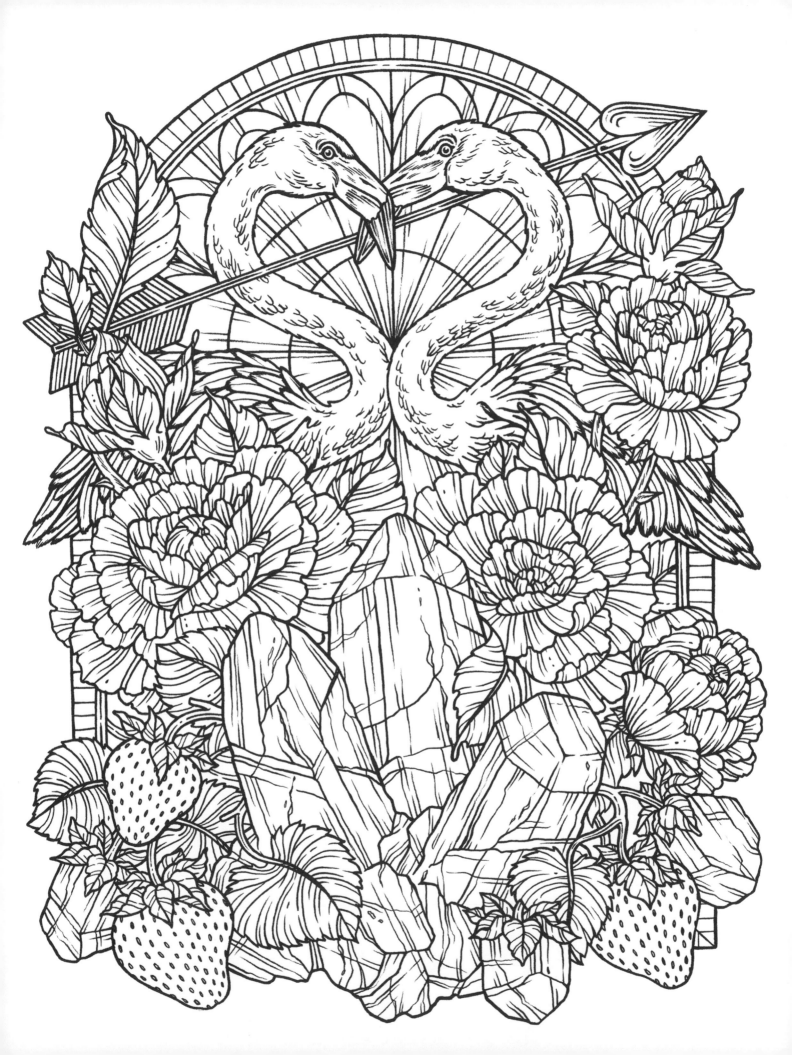

Tiger's Eye

With a captivating appearance that attests
its bold energies, tiger's eye displays shimmering
golden-yellow hues and is banded with stripes that
range from reddish-brown to inky black in color.
The polished stone emits a twinkling effect when light
is reflected from its surface, like that of a cat's eye.

Tiger's eye is a powerful protector, instilling in its
possessor the same spirit of strength, confidence, and
bravery as its namesake. In ancient Chinese lore,
tigers were seen as "spirit guardians" with deeply
protective powers, and tiger's eye was carved into
amulets and jewelry, used to shield the
wearer against evil spirits.

Associated with the solar plexus chakra, this gemstone's
sunshine hues and earthly powers bring about a deep
sense of determination and self-confidence. It helps the
user to live freely and fiercely, and guides them
towards finding their personal power.

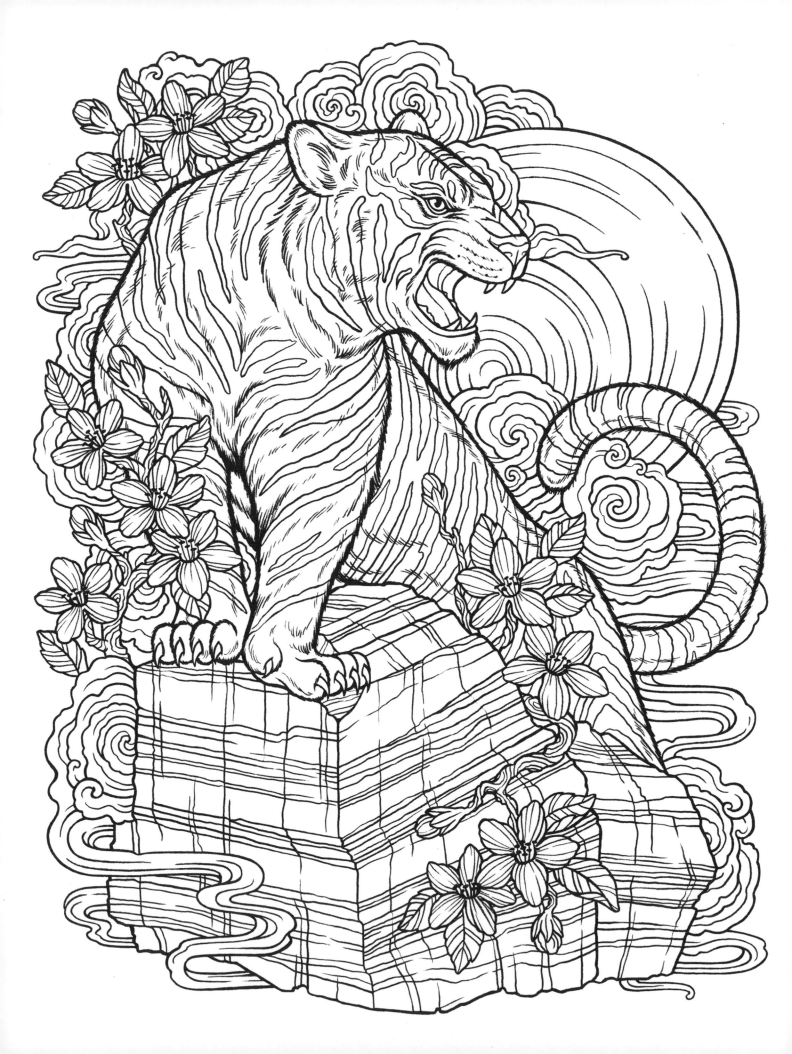

Blue Topaz

Blue topaz is a soothing gemstone of exceptional clarity. It has a calming glacier-blue color, ranging from soft pale blues to deeper shades. Associated with the throat chakra, it aids communication and encourages the possessor to speak confidently from an honest, open heart. A stone of compassion and empathy, it is thought to help with strengthening relationships and building bridges.

The peaceful scene of the lake and its reflection shown here evokes the same tranquility and balancing energies that blue topaz instills in its user. The bridge is symbolic of communication, connection, and stability. The crystal jutting out of the water, with its image mirrored below, represents the state of deep self-reflection and thoughtful meditation that blue topaz can bring.

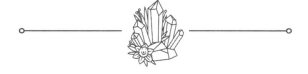

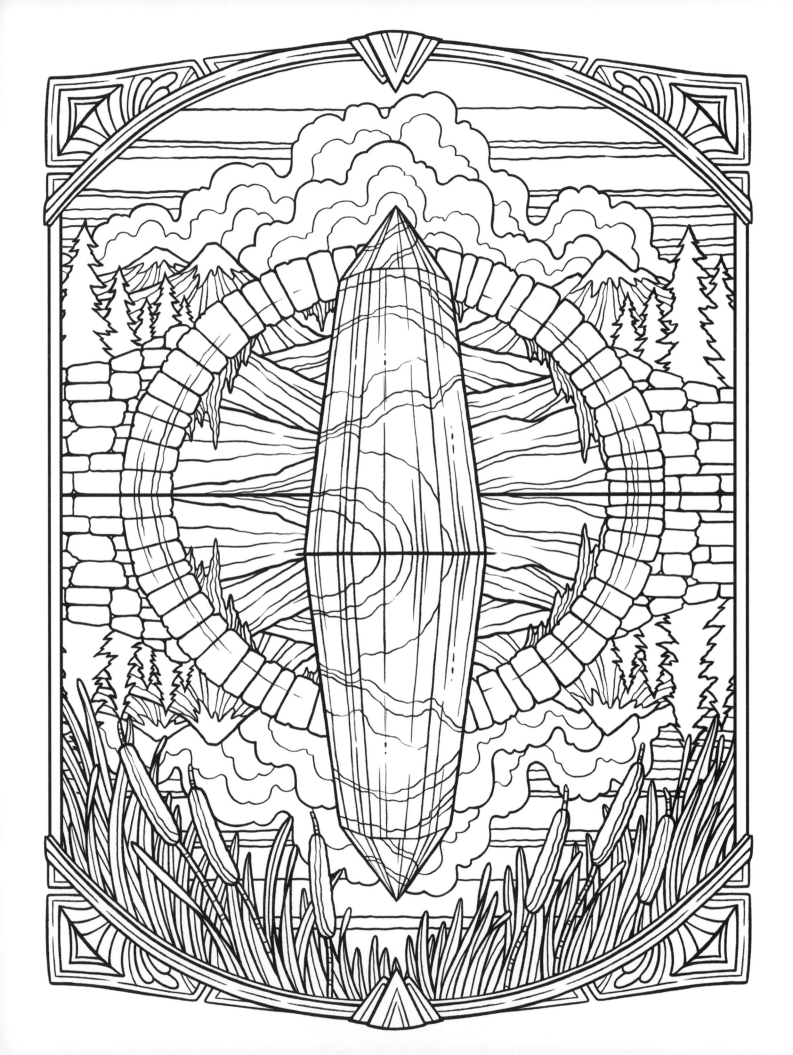

Agate

Agate comes in all the colors of the rainbow and has distinct, striped patterning. Each stone carries different healing properties and relates to a different chakra depending on the color. It has been prized since ancient times as a source of divine blessing. A powerful emotional healer, this harmonious crystal assists with communication, honesty, and unconditional love.

Like an anchor, agate helps to keep its possessor feeling grounded, focused, and connected to what matters most, by centering the mind and stabilizing the senses. The earthly energy and gentle nature of agate anchors the user to Mother Earth, bringing comfort and the ability to secure roots.

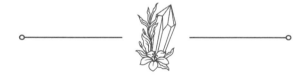

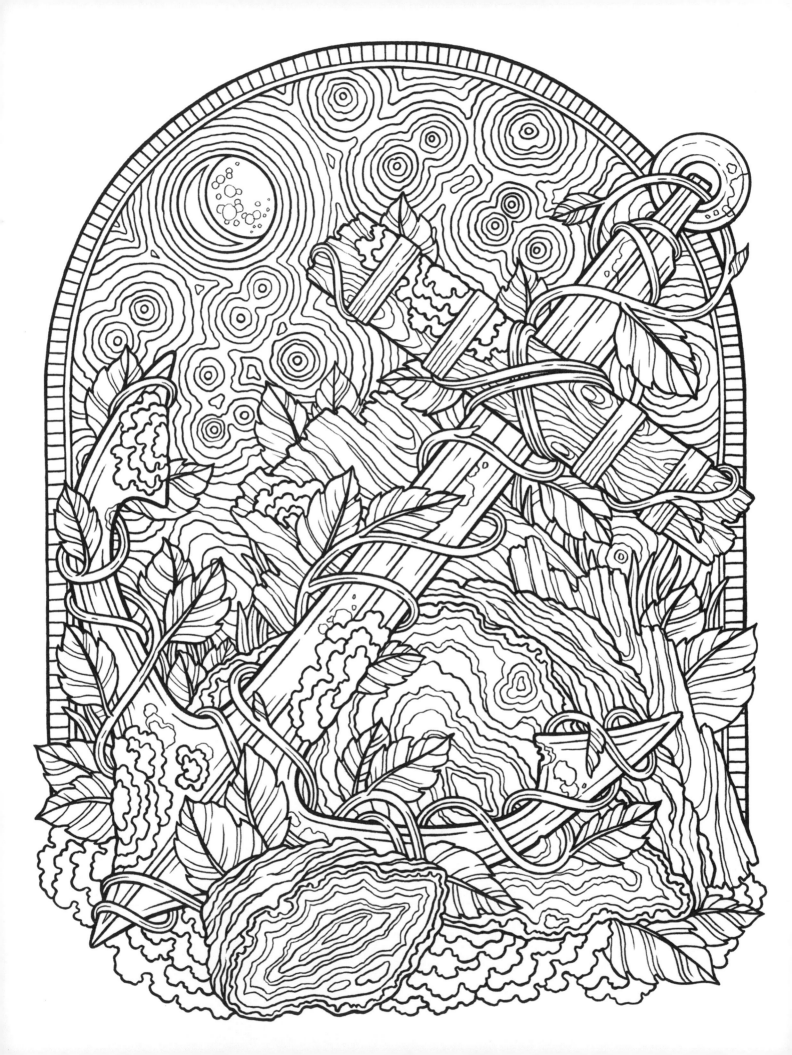

Opal

Bursting with amplifying energies, opal emits
high-frequency vibrations that are thought to activate
spiritual consciousness. It displays a unique opalescence,
causing a rainbow of colors to appear when light reflects
from its surface. These bewitching flashes, often referred
to as "fire," spark creativity and originality, while
promoting optimism and emotional harmony.

Opal is often used as a lucky charm, thought to
attract positivity and prosperity into the lives of those
who wear it. Koi fish are symbolic of these same virtues,
representing good fortune, strength, and perseverance.
They create a sense of perfect balance when swimming
in a pair, evoking the harmonious energies of
this mesmerizing gemstone.

A symbol of hope, purity, and truth, opal is essential
for those who want to harness its luminous "fire,"
ignite their inner confidence, and find inspiration.

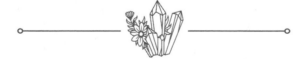

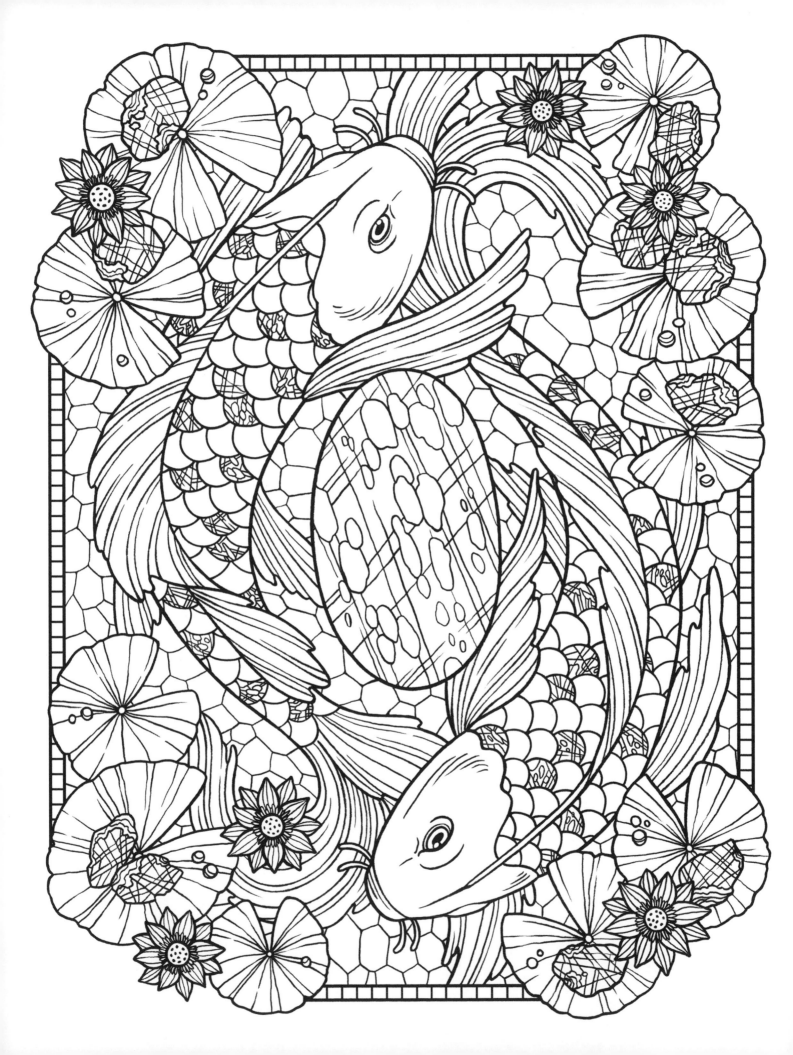

Spinel

A stone of revitalization and renewal, spinel is said to breathe a new lease of life into those who use it. With a strong connection to the Sun, its fiery orange-red color is associated with warmth, passion, and devotion.

Here, a majestic phoenix protectively clutches a spinel stone in its talons. The phoenix is known for its healing powers and has been a symbol of hope, transformation, and rebirth for thousands of years. It represents finding light in the darkness and rising from hardship with fresh life.

By stimulating the root chakra, spinel is said to increase physical stamina and vitality, helping to dispel stress and anxiety. It brings a bright optimism to those who want to revive their soul and feel reenergized, like a phoenix reborn from the ashes.

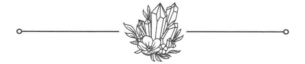

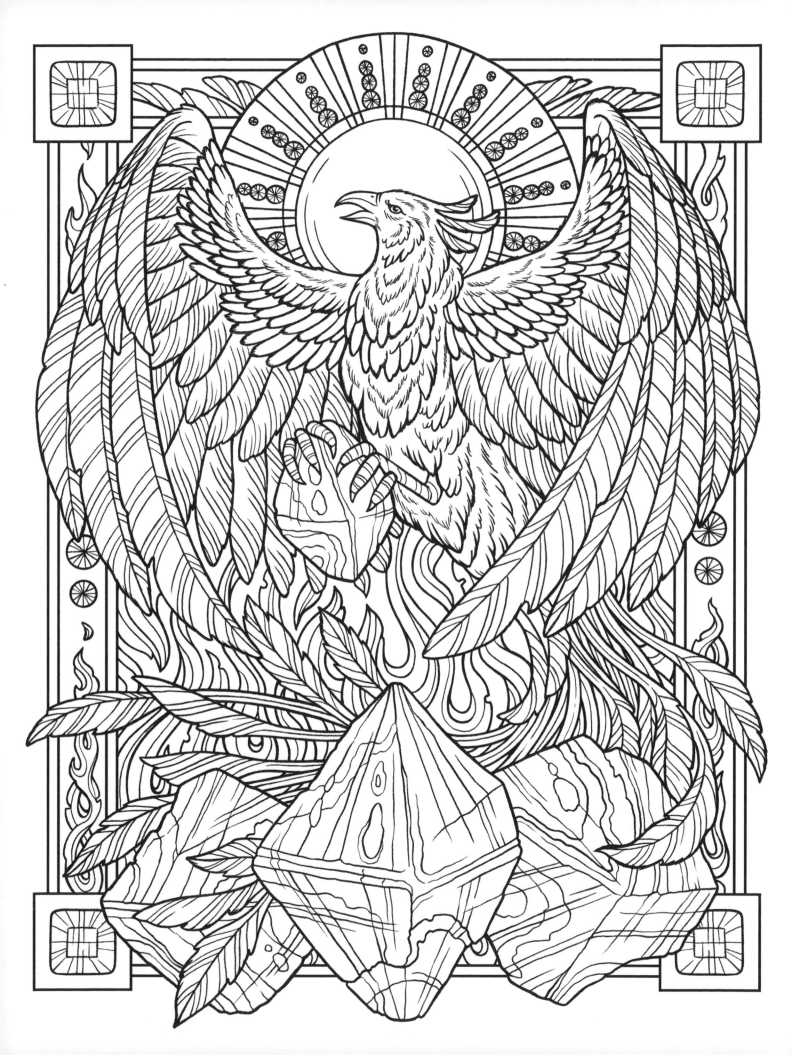

Labradorite

Labradorite is an empowering stone imbued with ancient magic and wisdom. It is often found in metallic shades of electric blue and forest green. Known for its spectacular displays of color, it flashes with bright-orange and copper-red hues when rotated in the light.

According to Inuit legend, labradorite provides a connection between our earthly plane and unseen, magical realms. It is inextricably linked to the aurora borealis, the phenomenal light show in the skies above the Earth's polar regions. Some legends say that the otherworldly lights are produced by Arctic "fire foxes," as their tails brush against the land and create sparks that light up the sky.

Labradorite helps the possessor find their inner light and tap into their own magical power, aiding connection to higher wisdom and truth. It is considered a powerful crystal for those who want to enhance their intuitive abilities and connections to the spirit world.

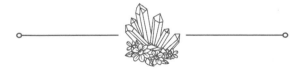

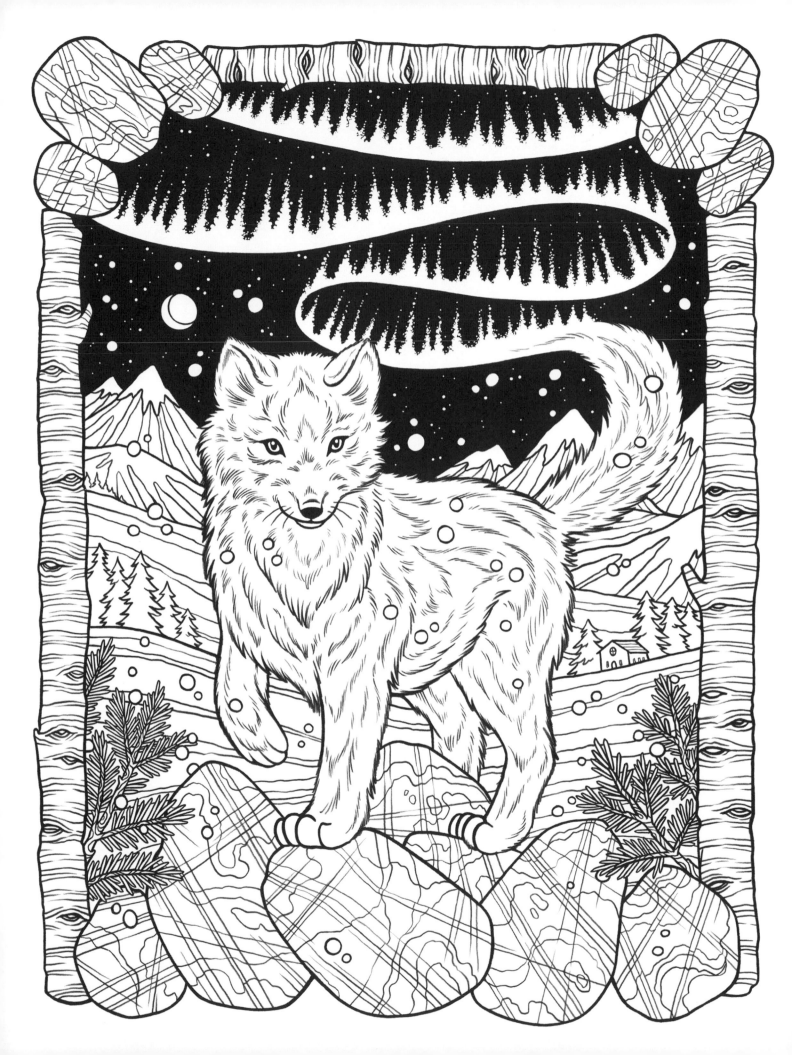

Peridot

A joyful stone with a deep connection to compassion
and kindness, peridot emits a warmth and radiant
shine that is sure to soothe, delight, and inspire. It has
been a symbol of wealth and opulence for thousands
of years. As a stone of the heart chakra, it is green
in color, coming in a range of glimmering hues
from a paler yellowish-green to deep olive green.

Here, peridot gems are interspersed among the
feathers of a peacock. Synonymous with the inner
radiance and prosperity this crystal provides, the
peacock's beautiful appearance and silky shine is
symbolic of wealth, power, and protection.

Peridot is a truly heart-focused stone, promoting
unconditional love and forgiveness. It is thought
to help heal past trauma. Its radiance uplifts the
spirit and cleanses the aura, bringing emotional
balance, growth, and happiness.

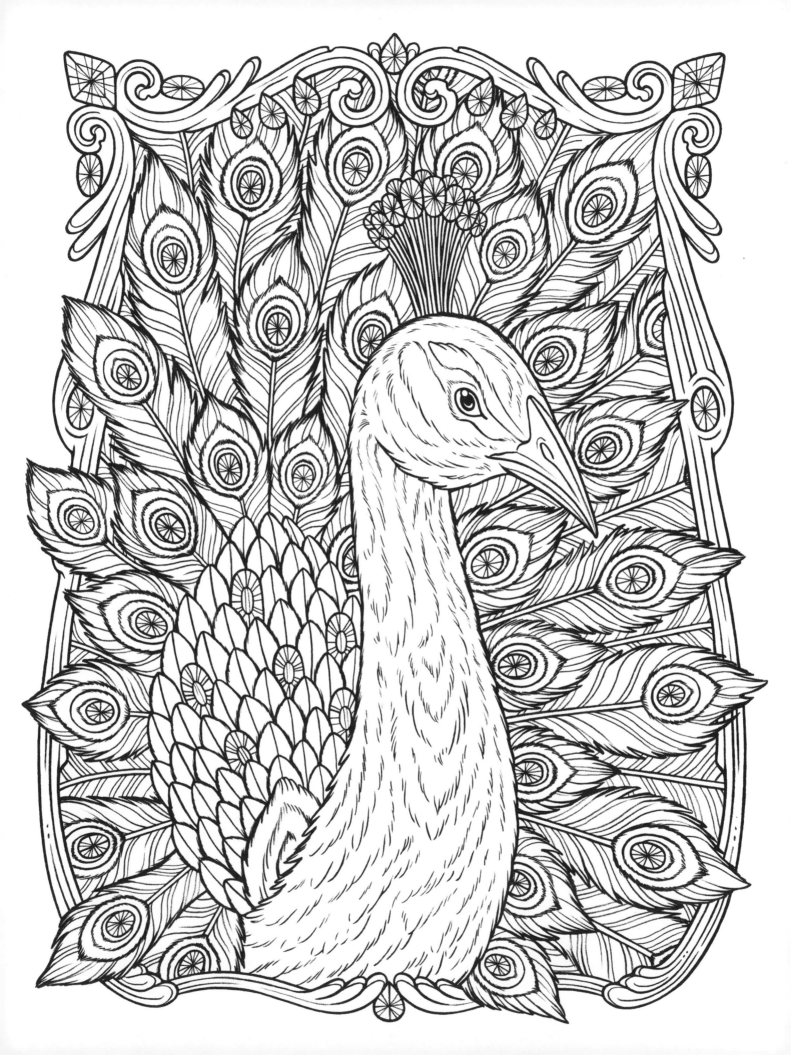

Moonstone

Ranging from pearly white to a spectrum of bright
blue, pink, and yellow hues, moonstone's changing colors
capture the mystical nature of a clear night sky. Soft and
silky in appearance with a shimmering iridescence,
it is thought to harvest the energy of the Moon.

Here, the gem is accompanied by moon flowers, which
bloom in the dark of night. Bats and luna moths are deeply
mysterious creatures, with a strong connection to the Moon
and its cycles, symbolizing transformation and rebirth,
much like this tranquil stone.

A protective stone that aids connections to higher
realms and enhances psychic intuition, moonstone
represents divine femininity and new beginnings.
Helping to balance emotions and embrace cyclical
change, this restorative stone is one of spiritual,
physical, and emotional healing.

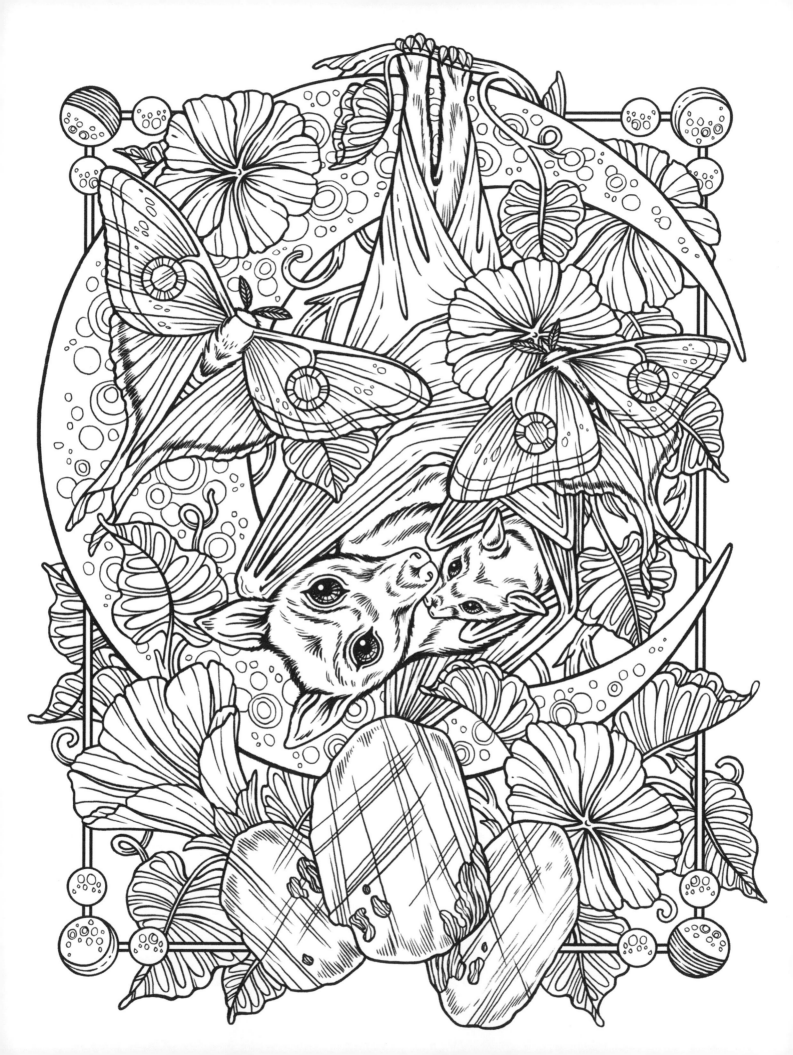

Bismuth

The crystal of transformation, bismuth is thought
to aid astral travel between the physical and spirit realms.
With a metallic appearance, it has a brilliant iridescence
in stunning multicolored shades, creating a feast for
the eyes in all the colors of the rainbow.

The healing energies of this crystal have the same
enriching effect on the spirit as its unique appearance
has on the eyes. Thought to connect the owner to their
higher self, bismuth is an excellent stone for enhancing
wisdom, insight, and greater knowledge.

It stimulates energy from the crown to the root
chakra through the whole body, helping the possessor
adapt to change and face challenges with confidence.
Teaching people to walk their own path in the cosmic
journey of life, bismuth facilitates achieving
goals and finding success.

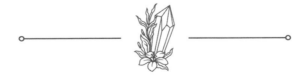

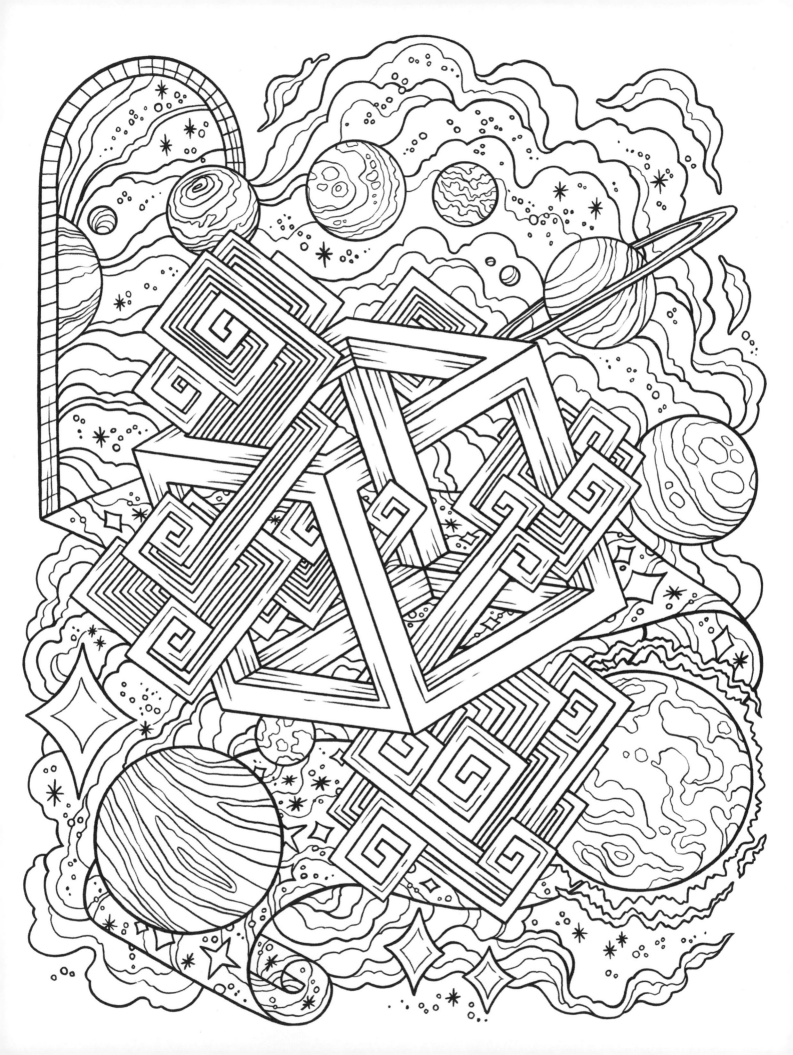

Sapphire

A stone of true celestial beauty, sapphire is
a precious gemstone that has, for centuries, served
as a symbol for the divine skies above. Sapphires
come in a range of beautiful hues, from pale blue
to deep azure and royal blues.

Symbolic of royalty, majesty, and nobility, the
vibrant sapphire gemstone has adorned kings, queens,
emperors, and rulers for thousands of years. Believed to
bring joy and clarity to its wearer, it is associated
with truth, loyalty, and wisdom.

Sapphire is connected to the throat and third eye
chakras, helping the wearer find their voice and follow
their intuition. Guiding them along their spiritual
path, it helps to activate a deeper level of
consciousness and spiritual connection.

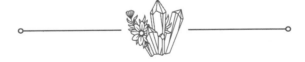

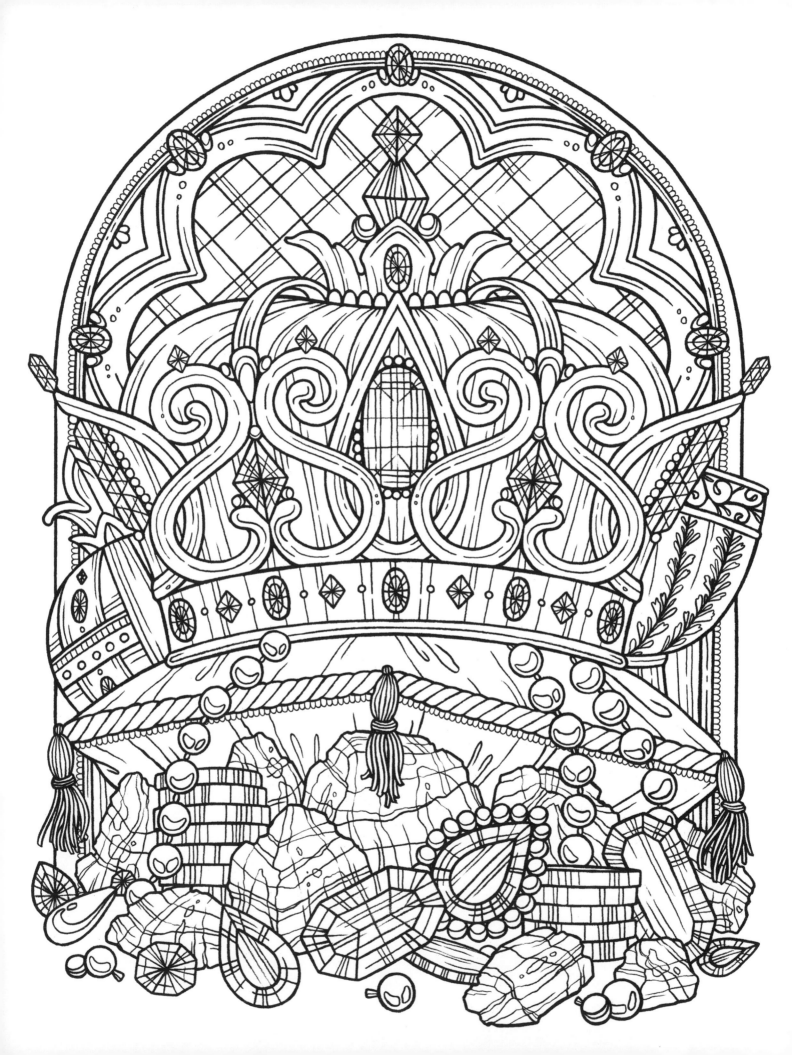

Ametrine

A rare and powerful stone, ametrine is said to bring balance by combining and amplifying the healing energies of amethyst and citrine. Merging deep-purple with golden-yellow hues, this crystal has a truly unique and beautiful appearance.

Ametrine is thought to give inner strength to those who use it. Associated with the crown and solar plexus chakras, it inspires tranquility of the mind, and can be used to boost positivity, motivation, and self-confidence.

Ametrine carries the harmonious energies of Yin and Yang and unites the divine masculine and feminine, allowing its user to find balance and be rid of emotional instability. Uniting two crystals together, ametrine instills a true sense of equilibrium in the mind, body, and spirit.

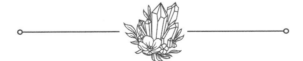

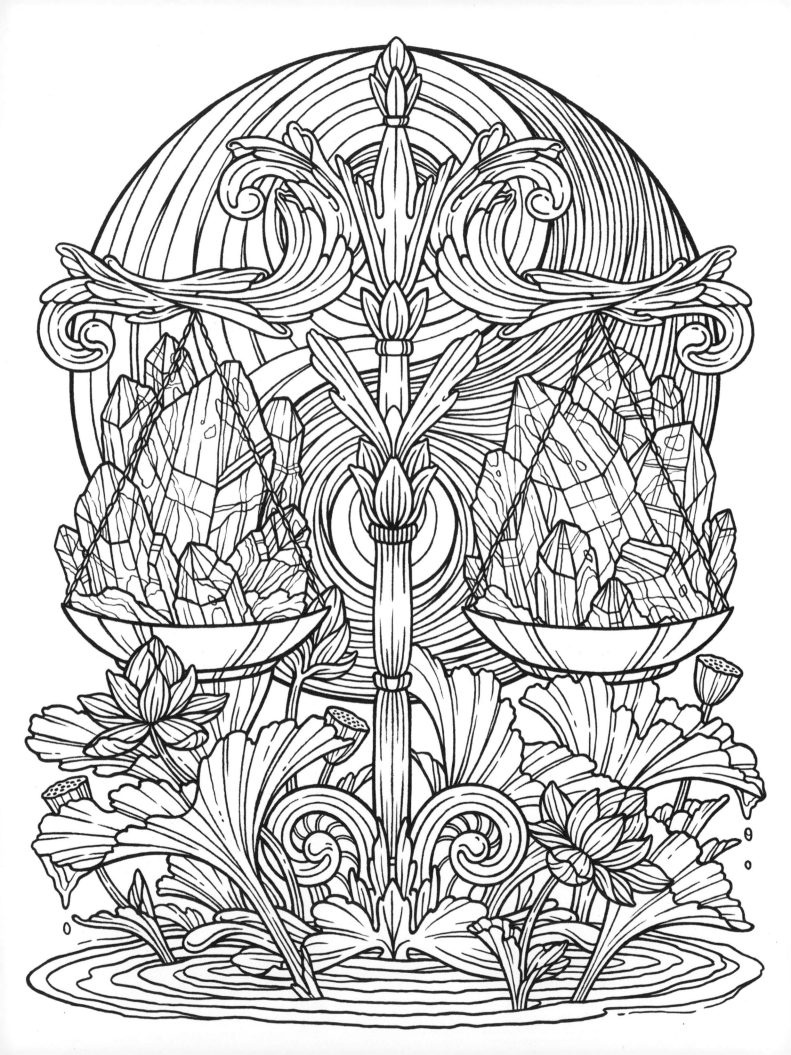

Larimar

The sea-blue hues of larimar, streaked with luminescent white lines, radiate the tranquility of crystal-clear waters rippling in the sunlight. Carrying the calming energies of gentle ocean waves, this crystal represents peace, clarity, and deep relaxation.

Known as the "Atlantis stone," larimar is believed to hold the ancient wisdom of the legendary sunken city. It is also sometimes referred to as the "dolphin stone," for its likeness to the animal's graceful and intelligent nature. Dolphins communicate on a high frequency, and this crystal, as a stone of the throat chakra, is celebrated for its ability to aid clear communication.

A powerful emotional cleanser, larimar is said to replenish the mind, body, and soul with the energy of the ocean. It promotes serenity in every aspect and encourages its possessor to live and love without fear.

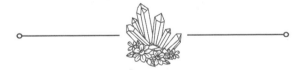

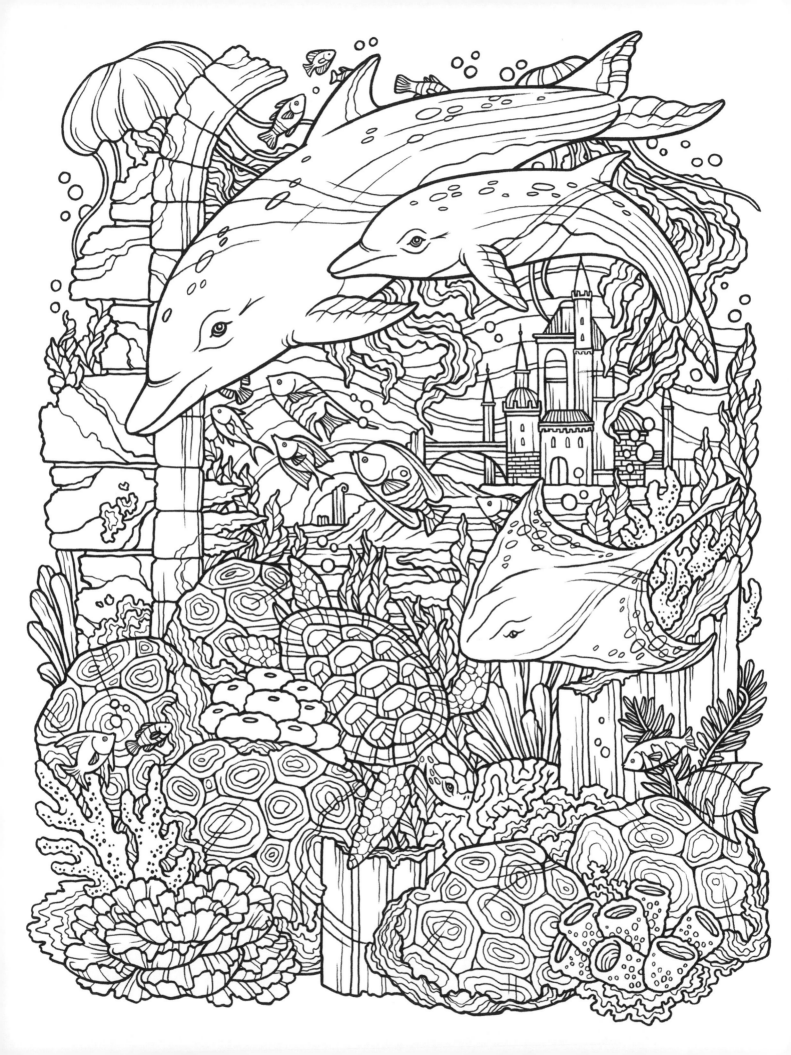

Alexandrite

Often referred to as "emerald by day, ruby by night,"
alexandrite is an extremely rare stone of exceptional
elegance and beauty. Its distinctive color-changing
ability makes it a truly magical stone, as it shifts from
shades of rich blue-greens under natural sunlight
to deep reddish-purples by candlelight.

Here, alexandrite crystals surround the planet Mercury,
as the stone is believed to be governed by the planet.
Mercury is named after the Roman god of the same name,
and it is said that the stone embodies the characteristics of
this ancient god, from hope, growth, and peace emanating
from its green appearance, to love, sensuality, and
passion from its red appearance.

The intertwining snakes are symbolic of wisdom and healing,
and this unique and extraordinary crystal is believed to hold
these same mystical qualities. It is believed to bring strength,
power, and prestige to those who possess it.

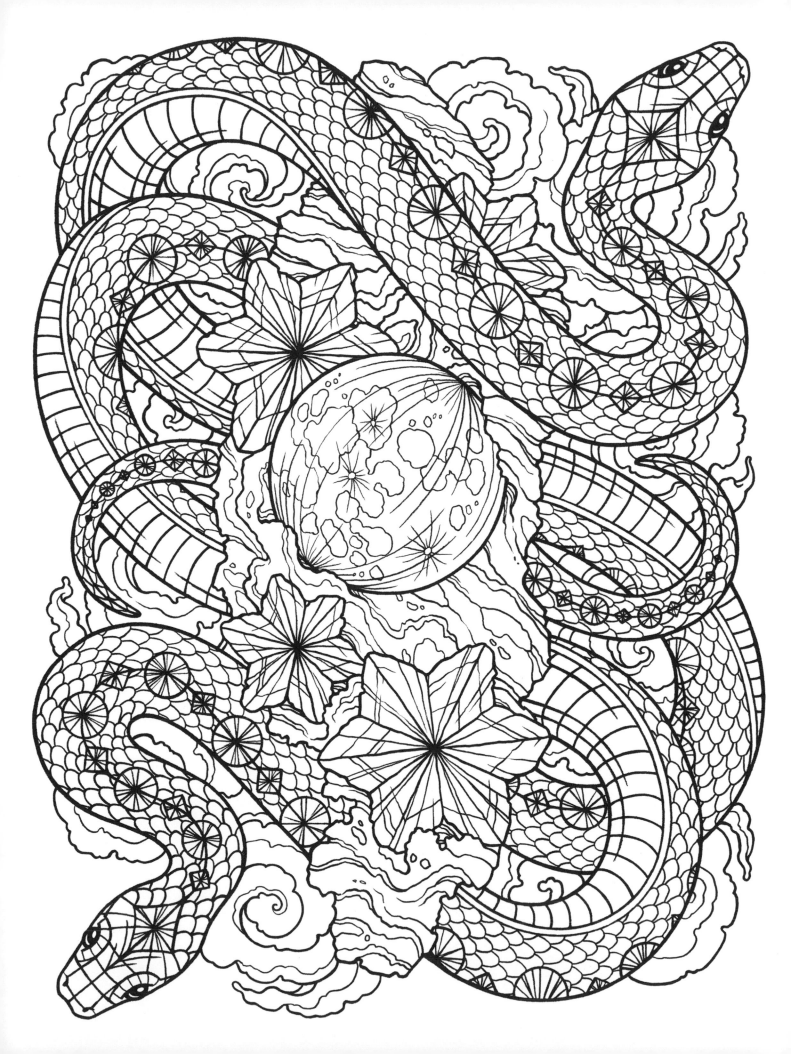

Carnelian

Like sunrise at the dawn of a new day,
the beautiful red-orange hues of carnelian represent
optimism and vitality. This energetic and positive crystal
is deeply associated with bravery and boldness, lending
courage to its possessor, and inspiring the strength
and power of a majestic lion.

Carnelian's rich, fiery color warms the spirit and
attracts the protective and passionate energies associated
with lions and fire. Believed to bring strength and
eloquence to the voice, carnelian has traditionally been
used to boost confidence and aid public speaking.

Energizing and empowering, yet with a strong
stabilizing and grounding force, this "sunset stone" helps
to reconnect the mind with the body and bring
passion and prosperity into the owner's life.

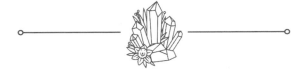

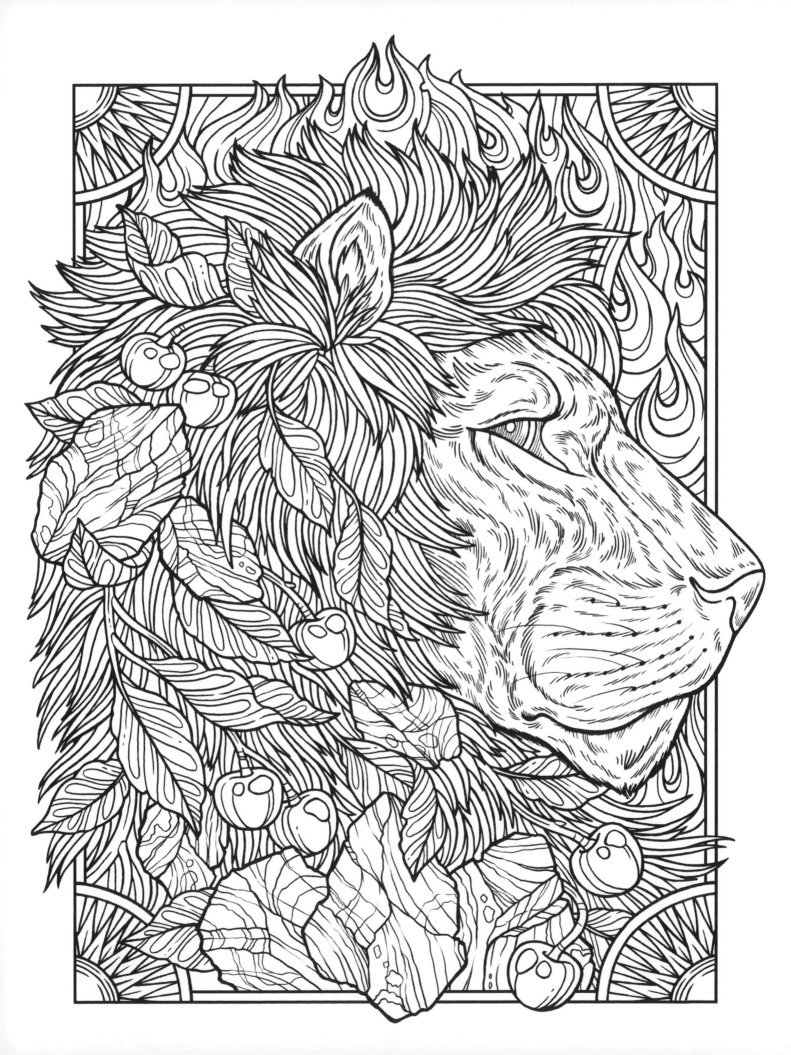

Pentagonite

Pentagonite is vivid blue in color with elongated blades of crystal extending from its center. Activating the third eye and crown chakras, it is believed to heighten psychic awareness and enhance channeling abilities by aiding communication with higher realms. Thought to inspire new ideas and drive away indecision, this crystal is all about the power of the mind.

Known as the "pentagram stone," pentagonite takes its name from the Greek word for five due to the five-pointed stars in its mineral structure, visible only under magnification. According to numerology, the number five represents freedom of spirit and embracing new beginnings.

Here, the crystal is pictured within an elemental pentagram carving. Each point represents one of the five elements in magical and occult beliefs—Fire, Water, Earth, Air, and Spirit. Together, they create a powerful symbol of life, protection, and balance.

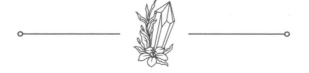

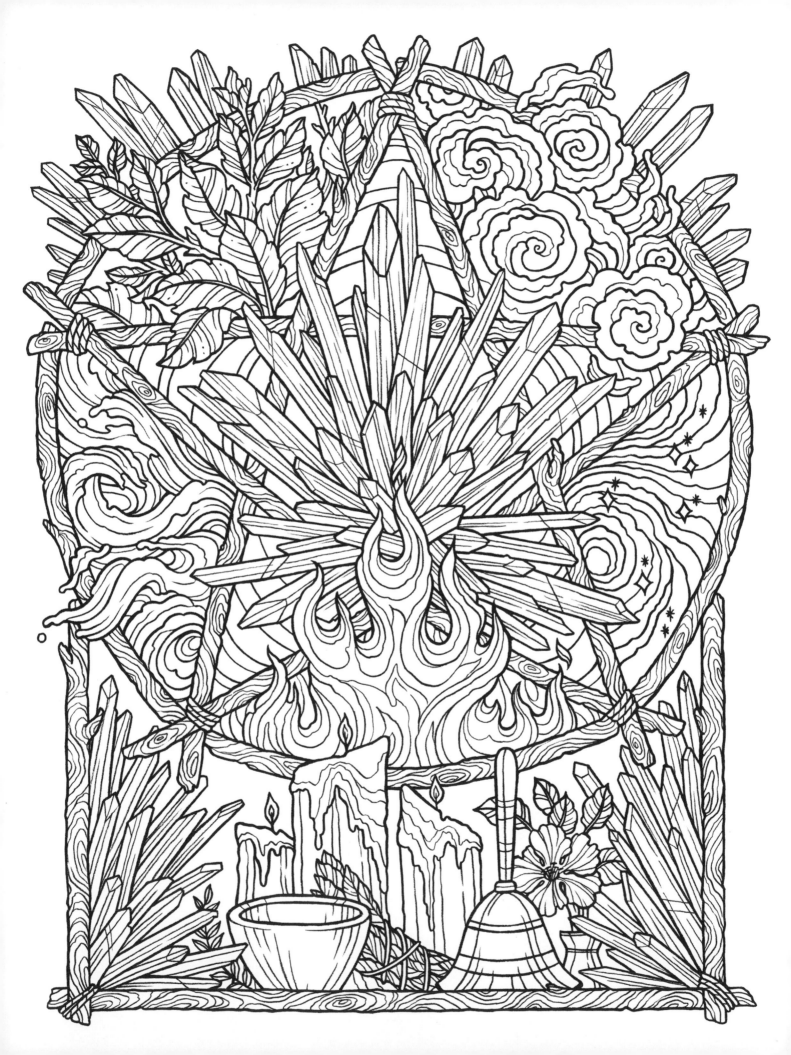

Diamond

Crystal-clear with a dazzling brilliance, diamond is unrivaled in the gemstone world. Known as the "stone of light," it has refractive powers causing light to diffuse into all the colors of the spectrum. This sparkling stone clears the shadows within, filling the soul instead with hope and optimism.

The icy scene here reflects the name "gem of winter" which is often ascribed to diamonds. Venus, which shines brightly in the night sky, is glimmering in the background, to show the gem's astrological association with the planet. With a strong connection to the Earth, the hare is symbolic of this magnificent gem's grounding energies of fertility and abundance.

Unparalleled in its hardness, diamond is sometimes referred to as the "stone of invincibility," and it is thought to encourage fearlessness and perseverance. Symbolic of purity and fidelity, it can bring everlasting love and clarity into relationships.

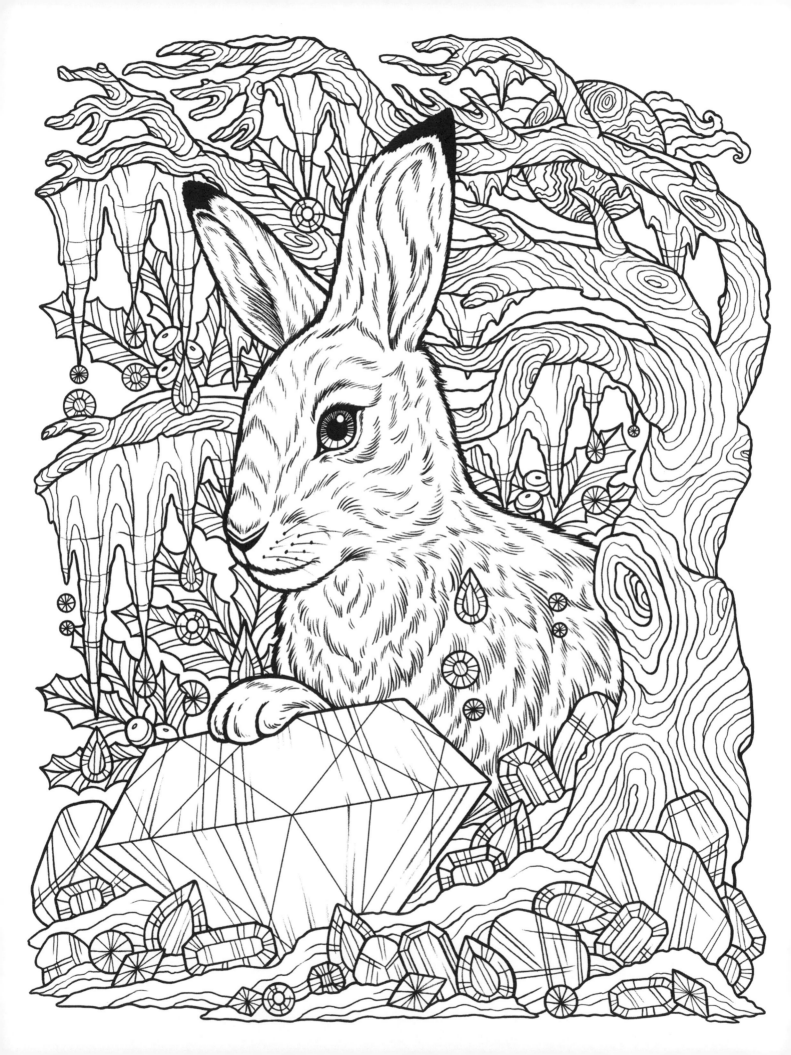

Lepidolite

Sometimes referred to as the "peace stone," lepidolite
is celebrated for its gentle nature and deeply nurturing
properties. Its soft, soothing lavender and lilac hues are
thought to have a calming effect on the mind, body,
and soul. A stone of gentle healing, lepidolite helps the
wearer break free from negative patterns to find
emotional stability and inner peace.

This balancing stone was named after the ancient
Greek word for scale, due to its reptilian texture and
scaly appearance. Chameleons are masters of adaptability,
changing their coloring to blend in and create harmony
with their environment. Lepidolite is also known as the
"stone of transition" for the stability it brings during times
of change, helping the user adapt and adjust to new
surroundings, just like a chameleon.

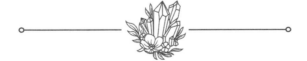

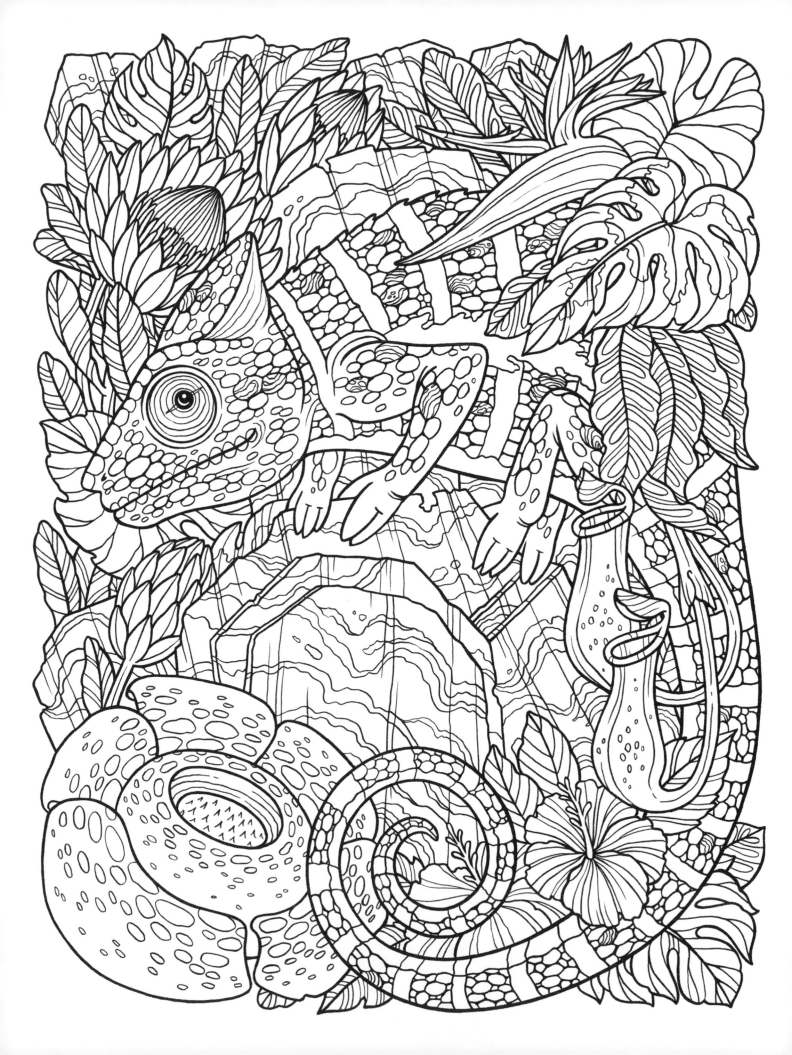

Vesuvianite

Also known as "idocrase," this crystal is commonly found in rich and earthy shades of green. A grounding stone that promotes stability and resilience, vesuvianite helps its user let go of fear and push away negative thoughts and emotions.

First discovered on Mount Vesuvius, this crystal is strongly linked to the divine realm and symbolizes moving forward and embracing change, like lava bursting from a volcano as liquid before solidifying into rock on the Earth's surface.

Vesuvianite's close connection to romance and the heart chakra makes it a common gift for newlyweds. Through boosting cooperation and communication with others, it is thought to aid in manifesting and fulfilling the heart's desires.

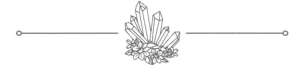

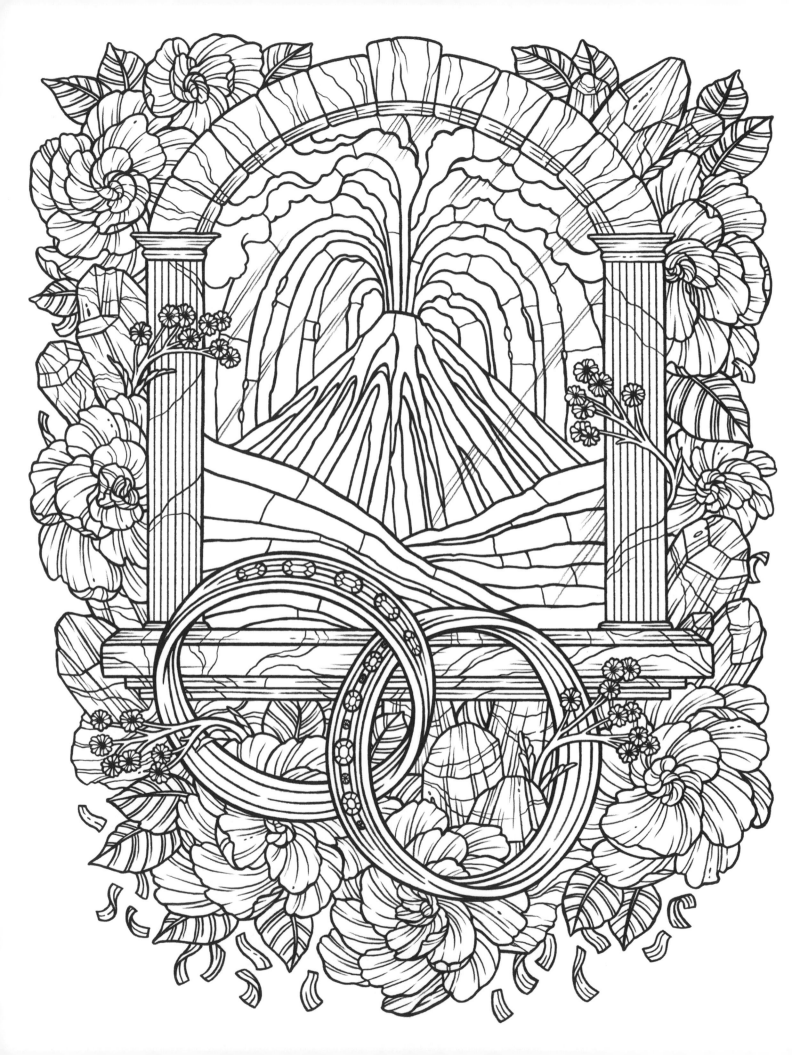

Red Phantom Quartz

Phantom quartz is a deeply healing crystal,
consisting of unique formations that are created by
interruptions in its growth, giving the appearance of
another crystal contained inside it. Red phantom quartz is
an extremely rare variety of quartz, which shows a clear red
phantom from an earlier stage of growth. Believed to restore
vitality and boost self-esteem, red phantom quartz inspires
creativity and is thought to help possessors achieve
their goals and deepest desires.

An excellent calming stone and emotional healer,
red phantom quartz enables possessors to feel grounded and
connected to the natural world around them. Thought to have
a special affinity with fairies and playful phantom creatures,
it can be used to help recover repressed memories and heal
the "inner child." Sometimes known as the "stone of
growth," it encourages the user to release stress
and let go of fear and worry.

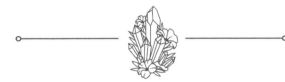

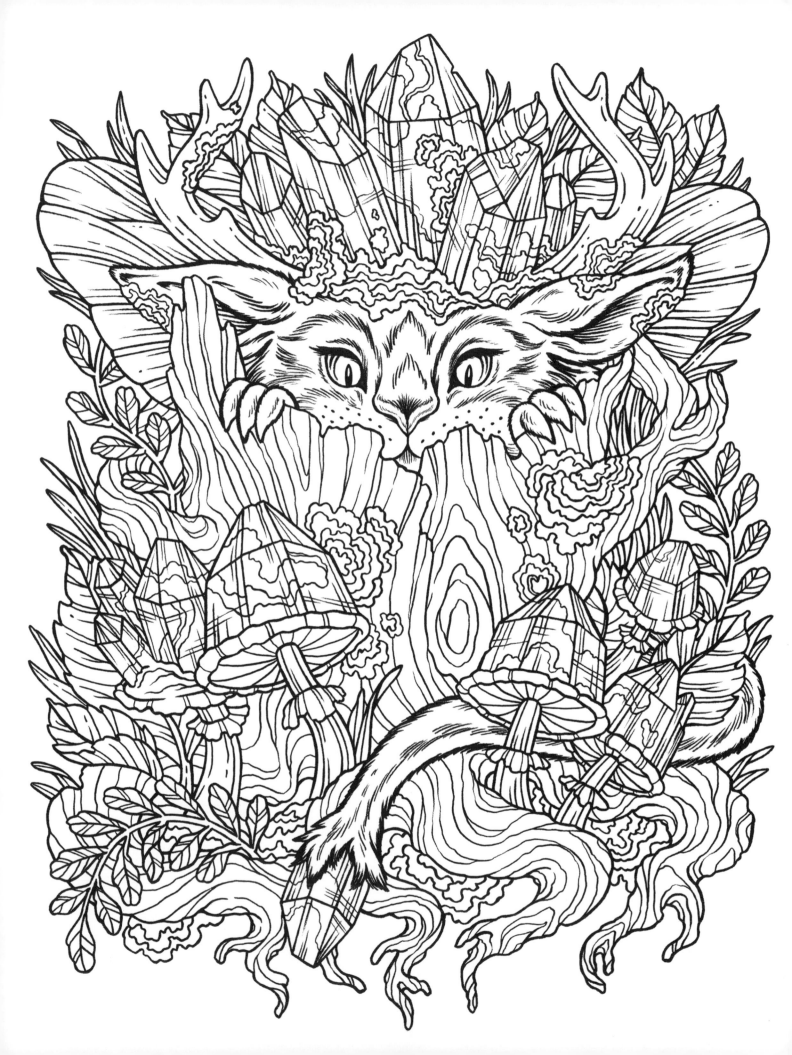

Lapis Lazuli

This semiprecious stone, with its energizing and vivid
deep-blue shades and flecks of pyrite gold, has been prized
throughout history for its close connection to the Divine.

In ancient Egypt, it was made into jewelry
thought to reflect the high status of its wearer. Used to
create ornaments and amulets, as well as the funeral masks
of pharaohs, this powerful stone was celebrated for its noble
and majestic associations. Here, it is depicted with
the Egyptian queen Cleopatra, who famously used
its bright-blue pigment as makeup.

Today, lapis lazuli is considered a crystal of wisdom
and truth, bringing physical and emotional strength and
spiritual intuition. By keeping this crystal close to the throat
chakra, the user can clear negative energies and freely
communicate the heart's deepest emotions.

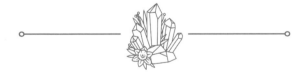

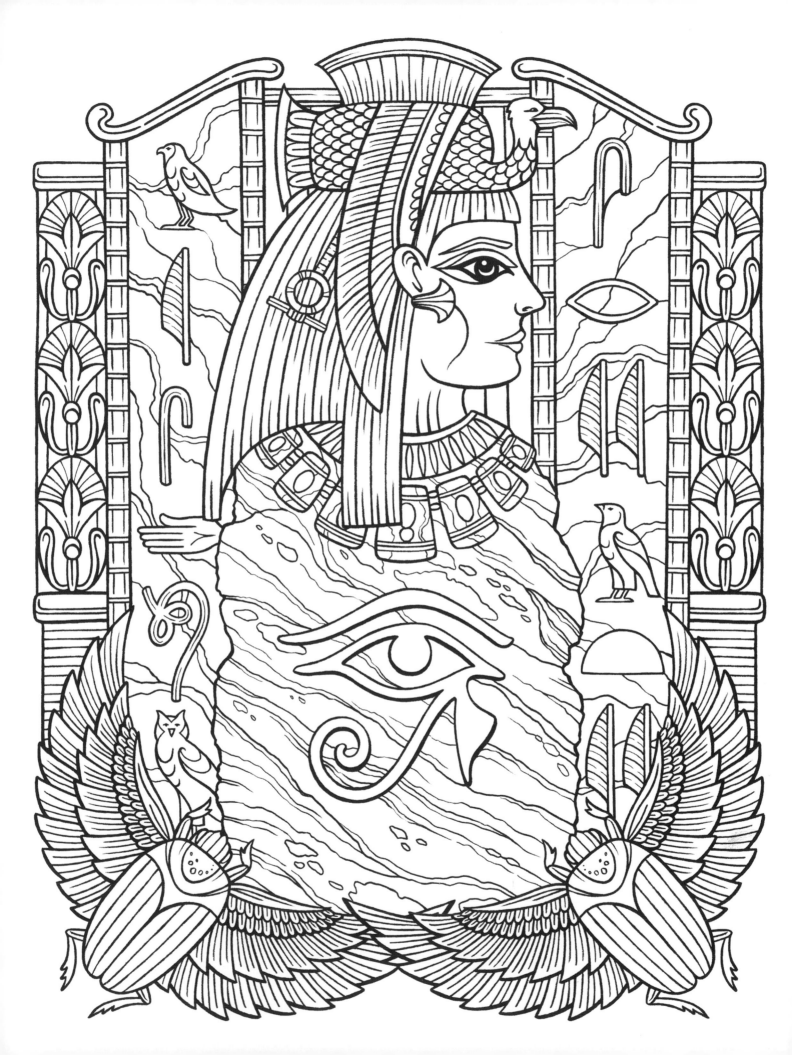

Bloodstone

Earthy green tones are peppered with bright flecks of bloodred crimson in this protective and striking stone. Bloodstone's connection to health and longevity spans thousands of years, and it has long been used as an amulet for courage and protection. Ancient warriors are said to have carried it into battle, believing it would stop the bleeding from their wounds, and protect them from the harm inflicted by the malicious glare of the "evil eye."

Symbolic of purification and justice, bloodstone is thought to bring strength. It helps to balance the body by realigning the lower chakras, keeping the wearer grounded. It has a strong connection to the elements and is believed to harness the power of the weather. Like a stormy sky giving way to sunshine, this long-beloved crystal has the power to banish negativity and bring hope in its place.

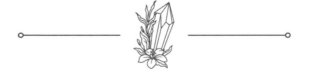

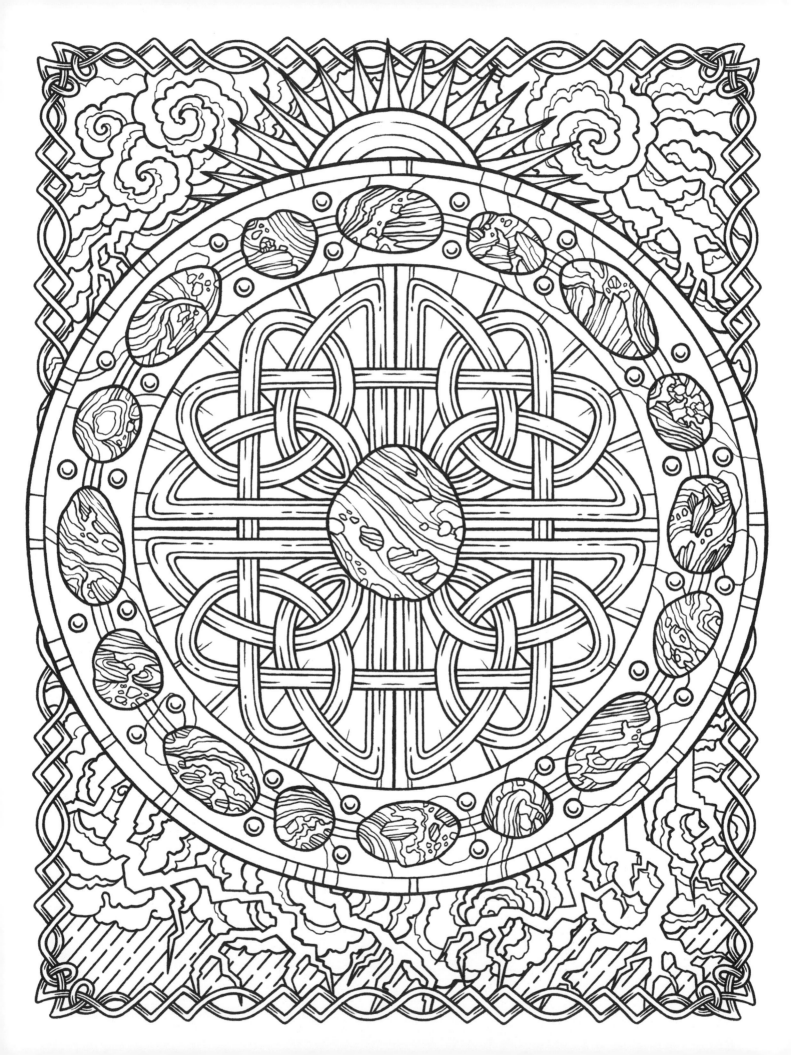

Garnet

Crimson in color, with deep-red hues, garnet has been a prized gemstone of passion for thousands of years. It is associated with blood and the heart, and fills the body with a protective and nourishing life force.

With its resemblance to pomegranate seeds, garnet has close associations with the mythological figure Persephone, who famously ate the seeds, condemning herself to spend half the year in the Underworld. According to the myth, this is how the seasons came to be, and the image here depicts each season, from the blossoming flowers of spring to the frosty branches of winter.

Known as the "commitment stone," garnet symbolizes everlasting love in friendships and romantic relationships. The locket shown here represents love and the things people hold dear to them, and garnet invites passionate energy to those who keep it close to their heart.

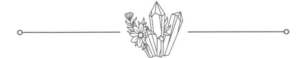

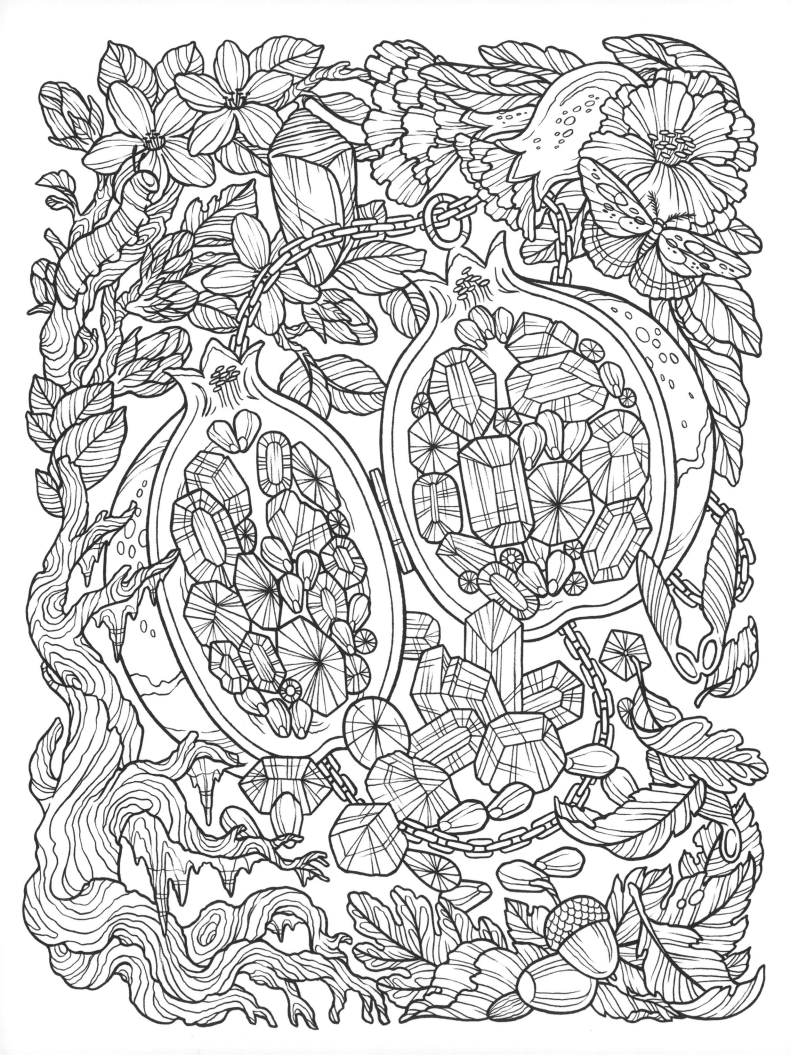

Sunstone

With a golden warmth and rich rosy glow, sunstone is said to harness its energy from the Sun. Promoting luck, joy, and happiness, it is believed to bring good fortune and positivity to the possessor, providing an invigorating burst of energy like bright Sun rays on a summer's day.

Sunstone was first discovered in the fjords of Norway and the Vikings are thought to have used it as a compass to navigate the seas. People still use the stone's bright energy and shimmering light as a source of spiritual guidance today.

A stone of the sacral and solar plexus chakras, sunstone facilitates creativity, independence, and confidence, helping to clear negative energy and allow a person's inner light to shine through.

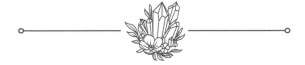

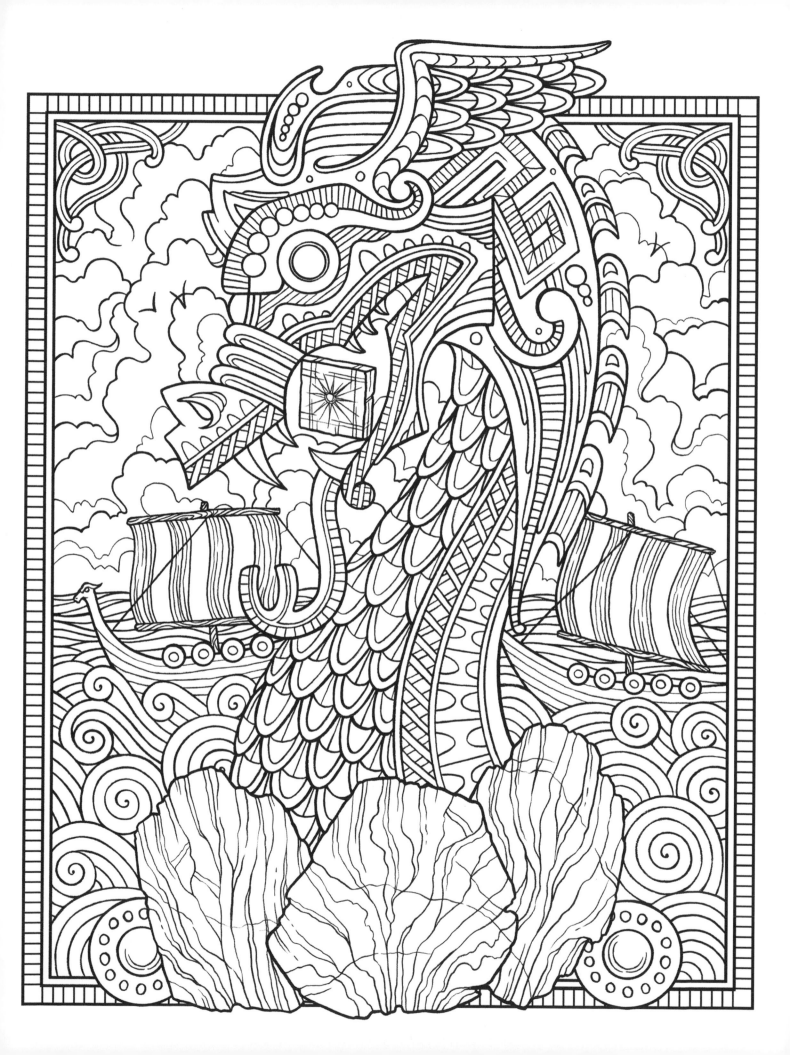

Moss Agate

Capturing the raw and timeless beauty of Mother Earth herself, moss agate is a clear crystal embedded with swirling, moss-like patterns in beautiful shades of deep forest green. The Gaia figure pictured here is carved from moss agate, and reflects the stone's beautiful appearance and soothing nature.

The crystal of gardeners and agriculture, moss agate has long been considered a lucky gemstone with the power to bring a prosperous harvest. Historically, farmers would hang the stone from tree branches and cattle horns in the hope it would harness the life-giving power of Mother Earth and bring them prosperity and wealth.

The spiritual meaning of moss agate is abundance, and its lush green coloring binds it to the heart chakra. With special balancing energies that soothe and uplift the soul, this is an essential crystal for those who want to feel grounded and connected to the world around them.

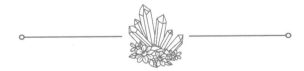

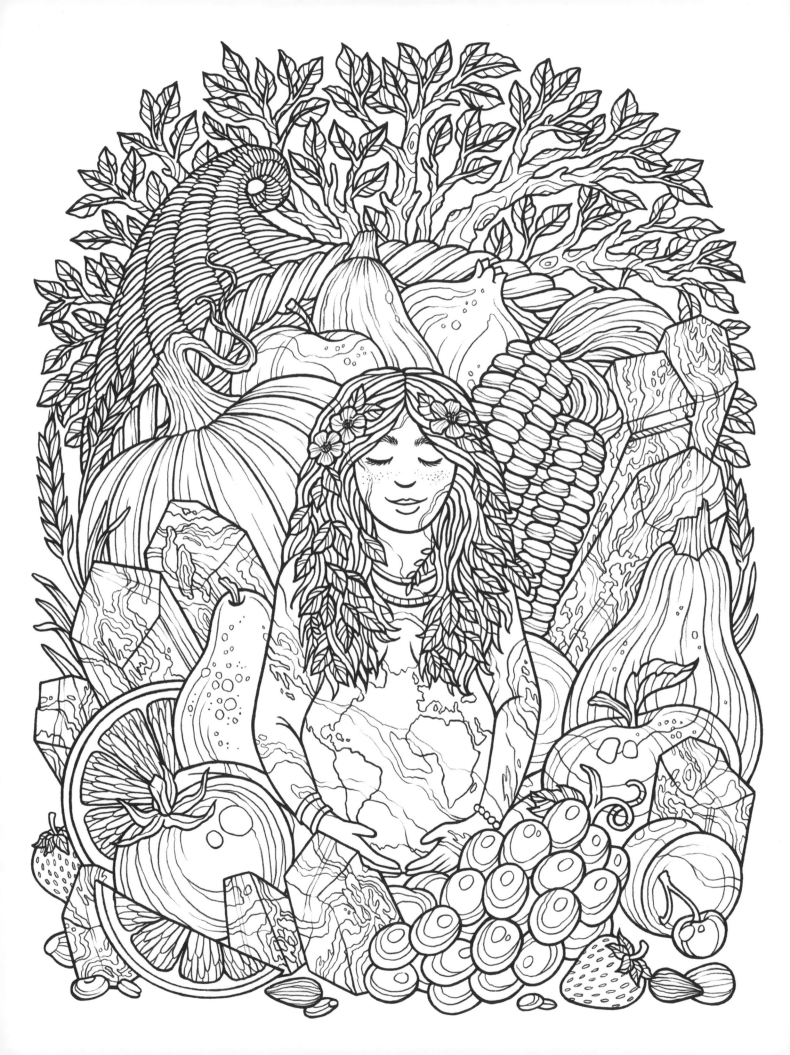

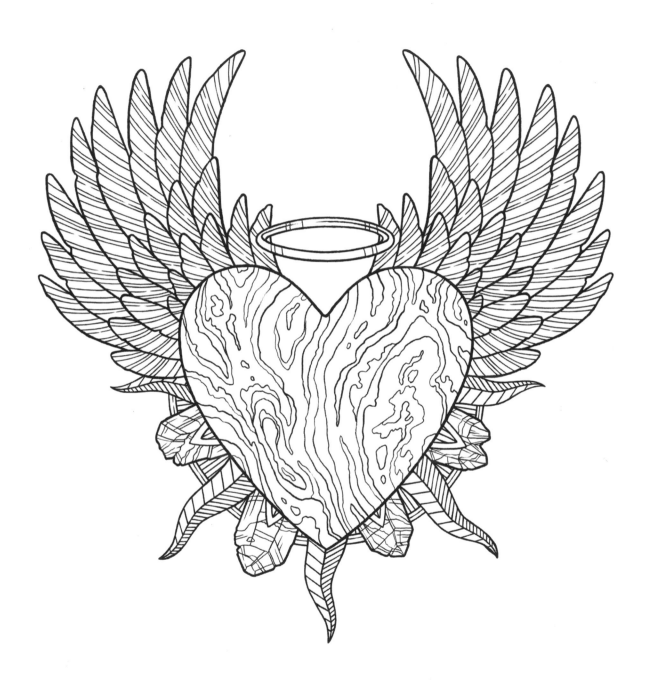